I ♥ SOUP

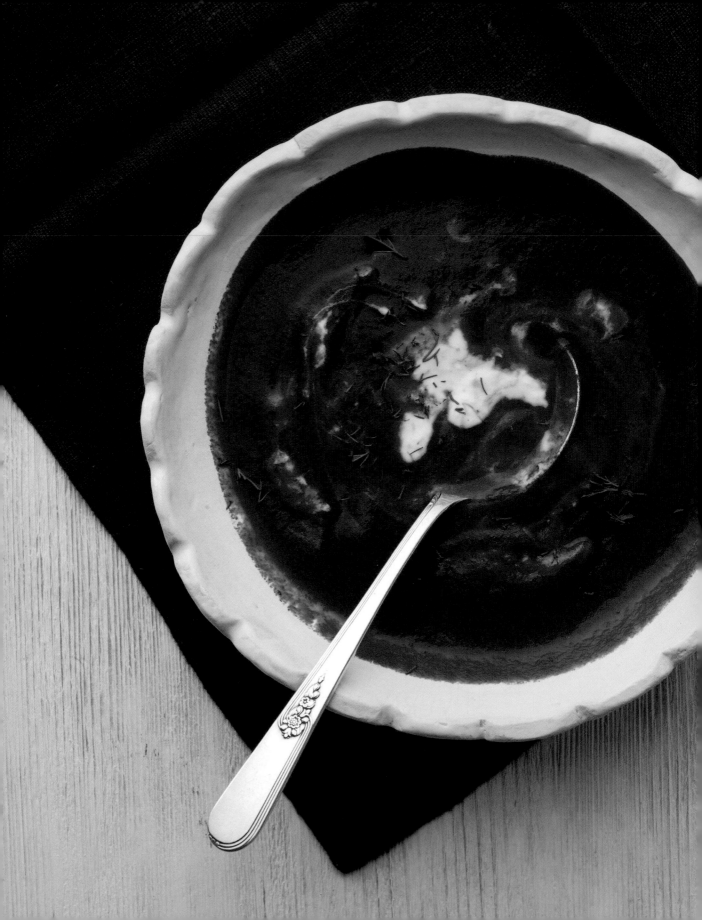

I ❤ SOUP

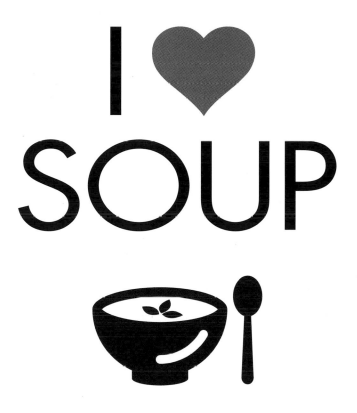

MORE THAN 100 OF THE WORLD'S MOST
DELICIOUS AND NUTRITIOUS RECIPES
FOR ALL SEASONS

BEVERLY LeBLANC

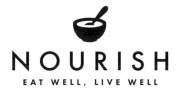

NOURISH

EAT WELL, LIVE WELL

First published in the UK and USA in 2016 by
Nourish, an imprint of Watkins Media Limited
19 Cecil Court
London WC2N 4EZ

enquiries@nourishbooks.com

Recipes taken from *The Big Book of Soups*, first
published by DBP in 2011

Managing Editor: Sarah Epton
Designer: Clare Thorpe
Commissioned photography: William Lingwood
Food Stylist: Bridget Sargeson
Assistant Food Stylist: Jack Sargeson
Prop Stylist: Lucy Harvey

A CIP record for this book is available from the
British Library

ISBN: 978-1-84899-764-6

10 9 8 7 6 5 4 3 2 1

Typeset in Adobe Garamond Pro and Futura

Colour reproduction by Scanhouse, Malaysia
Printed in China

Publisher's note
While every care has been taken in compiling the
recipes for this book, Watkins Media Limited, or any
other persons who have been involved in working
on this publication, cannot accept responsibility for
any errors or omissions, inadvertent or not, that may
be found in the recipes or text, nor for any problems
that may arise as a result of preparing one of these
recipes. If you are pregnant or breastfeeding or
have any special dietary requirements or medical
conditions, it is advisable to consult a medical
professional before following any of the recipes
contained in this book.

Notes on the recipes
Unless otherwise stated:
Use medium fruit and vegetables
Use medium (US large) organic or free-range eggs
Use fresh herbs, spices and chillies
Use granulated sugar (Americans can use ordinary
    granulated sugar when caster sugar is specified)
Do not mix metric, imperial and US cup measurements:
    1 tsp = 5ml 1 tbsp = 15ml 1 cup = 240ml
Flour for bread recipes should be weighed or
    scooped with a cup measure and then levelled:
    1 cup = 140g
All recipes serve 4–6
The symbols refer to the recipes only, not including
optional ingredients or serving suggestions. Check on
the packaging that all ingredients are dairy-, wheat-
or nut-free, or vegan, as brands can vary.

Symbol key
🍼 Dairy-free
🥜 Nut-free (coconut is being treated as a nut in this
    book, so recipes with coconut milk have not been
    labelled as nut-free)
🌾 Wheat-free
Ⓥ Vegetarian (no meat, game or seafood, but can
    contain dairy and egg products)
Ⓟ Vegan (no meat, game, seafood, dairy or egg
    products)

nourishbooks.com

CONTENTS

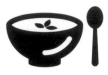

INTRODUCTION

As I spent several cold, grey winter months totally immersed in reading about, thinking about, writing about, making and eating soup, I came to appreciate how the universal popularity of soup comes not only from its ability to satisfy, warm and comfort, but also from its great versatility. The term 'soup' embraces many different liquid-based dishes, from thin, clear delicately flavoured broths to big steaming bowls of noodles, meat, poultry and vegetables. They can be righteously health conscious or indulgent, filling feasts-in-a-bowl. Consequently, whatever the time of the year and whatever the occasion there is always a suitable soup recipe.

As you work your way through this book, I'm sure you will soon appreciate how much soups have going for them. It doesn't matter if you are an accomplished family cook, or a bright young singleton juggling work and a hectic social life, you can make delicious soups. I believe mealtimes should be pleasurable whatever your time constraints, and soups provide quick-and-easy meals in a hurry or more substantial, satisfying repasts when time allows.

Supermarkets and fast-food outlets provide plenty of prepared soup options, but the case for making your own soups is unbeatable. From a straightforward financial perspective, you'll save lots of money. Many of the recipes in this book, for example, make 4–6 servings for less than the cost of a single pot of soup from my favourite deli. Although globalization gives us the opportunity to find virtually any ingredient all year round, the old adage that cooking with the seasons saves you money still holds true. Even if you are a devoted meat-eater, the Vegetable & Grain chapter offers plenty of scope for taking advantage of produce when it is most prolific and, therefore, least expensive. Soups also provide a wonderful way of transforming leftovers into a second meal, cutting down on waste, as well as your shopping bills.

The overriding benefit of getting into the habit of making soups on a regular basis, however, is that you can have exactly what you want, when you want it. Are you a champion of organic, free-range and sustainable farming? Choose your ingredients accordingly and it is easy to eat well following your principles.

If your main concern is to protect your family from ingesting the additives contained in processed foods, homemade soups are for you. To tempt fussy young eaters into getting a good mix of vegetables in their daily diet, try Golden Carrot & Sesame Soup (see page 135), or any of the farmers' market soups (see pages 119, 128–129 and 147), all of which adults will enjoy just as much.

Most of the recipes in this book can be cooked in large batches and frozen, making them perfect for lunches on the go. Many are complete meals in themselves, with a combination of protein and starch. You won't have to do much more cooking to ensure you eat a balanced meal. A bowl of soup with a hunk of good bread – and I've included recipes for several breads and rolls that even a novice can master – gives more than just the nutrients you need to get through the day, all for very little effort and very little expense.

The recipes make 4–6 servings (4 adult-size bowls, often with a little left for seconds, or 6 children-size portions). After you've made a few recipes, I'm sure you'll soon realize if you need to scale up or scale down the quantities for your requirements.

When I was planning this book I looked North, South, East and West for inspiration; the result is a mix of international flavours. This is a collection of my favourite soup recipes that I hope you will love as much as I loved writing them.

THE TECHNIQUES

Making stock for soups – Stock is the liquid that gives extra depth of flavour to many soups. It is perfectly possible to make delicious, satisfying bowls of soup without stock – the Aegean Red Mullet Soup (see page 90) and Oxtail Soup with Barley (see page 31) are two great examples – but most soups rely on stock for their final taste.

The quality of the stock you use determines the quality of your soup, and deciding which stock to use in a recipe is arguably the most important step of the process. You have several options, ranging from homemade stock to prepared fresh stocks from the supermarket, concentrated liquid stocks to be diluted with water, concentrated gelled stocks and powders and, finally, the ubiquitous stock/bouillon cube. The choice is personal, but least suitable is the stock/bouillon cube, because of its high salt content and metallic taste from the additives and preservatives. Using homemade stock, on the other hand, gives you total control over the quality of all the ingredients that go into your soup, but it is the most time-consuming option. This is why most recipes in this book specify a homemade stock or a ready-made option – the choice is yours.

Homemade stock is easily made by simmering meat, poultry or seafood bones and trimmings, vegetables and other flavourings, such as herbs and spices. The process extracts the colours, flavours and nutrients from the ingredients, all of which are then transferred to your soup. Stock-making can be a very enjoyable time in the kitchen. It is an undemanding task, and the result is satisfying. Once you've made a large pot of stock, you can also use it to flavour sauces and stews.

The stock recipes in this book make larger quantities than specified in most recipes. This is because stock can easily be frozen in portions, and once I've decided to make a homemade stock, I might as well make enough to freeze several portions. If you don't have much freezer space, leave the stock to simmer, uncovered, for longer until half the quantity is left, which will have a concentrated flavour. Then leave this rich, intensely flavoured liquid to cool completely and freeze it in ice cube trays. Use each cube straight from the freezer with enough cold water to complete 300ml/10½fl oz/1¼ cups of the stock specified in the recipe.

TOP TIPS FOR TOP STOCKS

- 'Take stock and then make stock' is sage advice. Stock-making is a good way to utilize vegetables past their prime but not yet ready for the compost bin. Vegetable trimmings, such as mushroom trimmings, tomato skins and onion skins (which give stock a richer, golden brown colour) are also excellent additions. Do not, however, include rotten or mouldy vegetables.
- Do not include potatoes in stocks because they make the liquid cloudy.
- Always break or chop bones before using them in stock. This gives the finished stock its slightly gelatinous texture that elevates soups made with homemade stock above ready-made versions.
- Trimmings from flat fish, such as plaice/flounder or sole, make excellent stock. Ask a fishmonger for these. They will likely be free or very inexpensive. Do not, however, include bones, heads or trimmings from oily fish in fish stocks.

- If you don't have time to make stock after roasting a chicken or large piece of beef on the bone, freeze the bones. Also freeze fish heads, bones and trimmings, and prawn/shrimp shells.
- Never let a fish, meat or poultry stock boil, or it will turn cloudy.
- Take care not to over-season stocks or your soup will be too salty. Use only a small amount of salt at the beginning of cooking to draw out the flavour of the other ingredients. Do not season it again. This is especially important if you intend to reduce the stock before freezing.
- Add the flavouring ingredients, such as chopped vegetables, herbs and spices, after you have finished skimming the surface.

Skimming soups and stocks – Stocks cook largely unattended, but your attention is most required toward the beginning of the process. As meat, seafood or poultry bones and trimmings are slowly heated to just below the boil, impurities are released and a grey scum appears on the surface. Use a large metal spoon, a slotted spoon or a round, perforated skimmer to remove this scum from the surface and discard it before adding the other flavouring ingredients. Take care not to remove too much of the liquid. Skimming can be a slow process, taking up to 30 minutes, but after you've finished this step you can leave the stock to gently simmer on its own. Pulses/legumes and vegetables also give off impurities while they simmer, but it isn't necessary to remove these. After you purée pulses, however, the thick layer of 'foam' that rises to the surface should be removed.

Storing stocks – Stocks are ready to use immediately after cooking. Alternatively, leave them to cool completely, then cover and refrigerate for up to 2 days or freeze for up to 6 months.

Adding flavour to soups with cheese rinds and ham hocks – Use natural hard cheese rinds to add an intense but subtle flavour to slowly simmered soups. Simply scrub off any markings, wrap them in cling film/plastic wrap and freeze them until you're ready to use them.

Add a piece of rind to your soup and simmer for anywhere from 10 minutes to several hours – the longer the rind simmers the more likely it is to totally dissolve into the soup. When ready to serve the soup, use a slotted spoon to fish out the soft rind, and either discard it or cut it into small pieces to sprinkle over the soup. Parmesan, pecorino, mature Cheddar and any other hard cheese with a natural rind all work well. Do not use wax-covered rinds.

The end of a Parma/prosciutto or Serrano ham also contains lots of flavour, even if not enough meat for cooks to bother slicing. They can be used to add 'meatiness' to soups without the expense. You will find these at meat counters and delis, and often you will be given them for free. After gentle simmering, remove the meat from the rind and any bones and finely shred it over the soup. Most cheese rinds and ham hocks are salty, so don't add extra salt until the end of the cooking process.

Making a bouquet garni – A bouquet garni is a bundle of fresh herbs, and often other ingredients, used to flavour soups. Tying the herbs together in a 'bouquet' with a piece of string makes it easier to remove them at the end of cooking. Always lightly crush the herb stalks with the back of a knife because they usually have more flavour than the leaves. If you don't have fresh herbs available, put dried herbs in a square of muslin/cheesecloth and use a piece of string to secure it closed.

Chargrilling, roasting and peeling peppers – To chargrill peppers, preheat the grill/broiler to high and lightly grease the grill/broiler rack. Halve the peppers lengthways and remove the cores and seeds. Put the peppers, cut-sides down, on the grill/broiler rack and grill/broil until lightly charred. Transfer to a bowl, cover with a clean, folded dish towel and leave to cool, then peel.

To roast peppers, preheat the oven to 220°C/425°F/Gas 7. Prepare the peppers as above, put them in a baking dish and roast for 40–45 minutes until lightly charred. Remove from the oven and prepare for peeling as above.

Peeling, deseeding and grating tomatoes – Cut a small cross in the bottom of each tomato using a sharp knife, put them in a heatproof bowl and cover with boiling water. Leave to stand for 2–3 minutes, then drain. Use a small knife to peel off the skins and discard them. To deseed the tomato, cut it in half lengthways and use a small spoon to scoop out the core and seeds.

A quicker way to peel tomatoes is to grate them on the coarse side of a box grater, pressing firmly, and then discard the skin and core. The disadvantage, however, is that the tomato pulp will also include all the seeds.

Toasting nuts and seeds – Toasting gives nuts and seeds a deeper flavour. Heat a dry frying pan over a high heat until hot. Arrange the nuts or seeds in a single layer and dry-fry, stirring continuously, for about 2 minutes until they start turning golden and you can smell the aroma. Immediately transfer to a plate to prevent them from overbrowning or burning. Toasted nuts and seeds can be stored in airtight containers in a dark cupboard for up to 3 months.

Judicious seasoning – You can always add extra seasoning, but it's very difficult to mask the flavour of too much seasoning. Most of the recipes in this book season at an initial stage of cooking to draw out the flavours of the ingredients. Do this very lightly because you will adjust the salt and pepper again before serving. Always cook potatoes and rice in salted water, but season dried pulses/legumes after cooking so the salt doesn't draw out the moisture acquired during soaking.

If you accidentally over-season a soup, add a little sugar or, if suitable, boil a peeled and chopped floury/russet potato in the soup. Taste soups before puréeing – you can always discard half the stock and replace it with fresh, unseasoned stock for a less salty taste, if necessary, at that point.

BASIC RECIPES

BEEF STOCK

MAKES about 2l/70fl oz/2 quarts
PREPARATION TIME 15 minutes, plus overnight
   chilling (optional)
COOKING TIME 7 hours

2.5kg/5½lb beef bones, chopped into large pieces
   (ask the butcher to do this)
3 large unpeeled onions, quartered
3 carrots, coarsely chopped
2 celery stalks, coarsely chopped
4 large garlic cloves, lightly crushed
1 bouquet garni made with 1 bay leaf and several
   parsley and thyme sprigs tied together
1 tbsp tomato purée/paste
12 black peppercorns, lightly crushed
a small pinch of salt

Preheat the oven to 230°C/450°F/Gas 8. Put the
bones in a heavy based roasting pan and roast for
50 minutes–1 hour until browned all over.

Stir in the onions, carrots and celery and roast for
another 30–40 minutes until the vegetables are very
tender and browned. Watch closely so they do not burn.

Transfer the bones and vegetables to a heavy stockpot
and add 4.5l/157fl oz/4½ quarts water. Bring to the
boil, uncovered, over a high heat, skimming the surface.
This can take up to 20 minutes. When the foam stops
rising, add the remaining ingredients, reduce the heat
to very low (use a heat diffuser if you have one) and
simmer, covered, for 5 hours. Do not let the liquid boil.
Skim the surface occasionally, if necessary.

Very carefully strain the stock through a muslin-lined/
cheesecloth-lined colander into a large bowl and
discard all the flavourings. Skim any fat from the surface
and use immediately. Alternatively, leave the stock to

cool completely, then cover and refrigerate overnight.
The next day, use a large metal spoon to 'scrape' the
congealed fat off the surface. Once cool, the stock will
be lightly gelled. See page 9 for storage information.

RICH CHICKEN STOCK

MAKES about 2l/70fl oz/2 quarts
PREPARATION TIME 15 minutes, plus overnight
   chilling (optional)
COOKING TIME 2½ hours

2 celery stalks, with the leaves, coarsely chopped
1 large carrot, peeled and chopped
1 large onion, peeled but left whole
1 bouquet garni made with 2 bay leaves and several
   parsley and thyme sprigs tied together
1 chicken, about 1.5kg/3½lb
6 black peppercorns, lightly crushed
a small pinch of salt

Put the celery, carrot, onion, bouquet garni and
1.5l/52fl oz/6½ cups water in a stockpot. Cover
and bring to the boil. Skim, then add the remaining
ingredients and 1l/35fl oz/4½ cups water, or enough
to cover the chicken. Bring the liquid to just below the
boil, skimming the surface as necessary. Do not let the
liquid boil.

Reduce the heat to very low, cover and simmer for
1¾–2¼ hours until the meat almost falls off the bones.

Remove the chicken from the pot and set aside for
another use. Strain the stock into a bowl and discard
the flavourings. Skim the fat from the surface and use
immediately. Alternatively, leave the stock to cool
completely, then cover and refrigerate overnight. The
next day, use a large metal spoon to 'scrape' the
congealed fat off the surface. Once cooled, it will be
slightly gelled. See page 9 for storage information.

CHICKEN STOCK

MAKES about 2l/70fl oz/2 quarts
PREPARATION TIME 10 minutes
COOKING TIME 3¼ hours

carcass and bones of 1 cooked chicken, or 900g/2lb
    mixed chicken bones, chopped
1 carrot, peeled and sliced
1 celery stalk, with the leaves, sliced
1 bouquet garni made with 1 bay leaf and several
    parsley and thyme sprigs tied together
6 black peppercorns, slightly crushed
a small pinch of salt

Put the chicken and 2.5l/88fl oz/2½ quarts water in
a heavy stockpot. Bring to just below the boil, skimming
the surface as necessary. When the foam has stopped
rising, add the remaining ingredients, reduce the heat
to very low (use a heat diffuser if you have one) and
simmer, covered, for 3 hours. Do not let the liquid boil.
Skim the surface occasionally, if necessary.

Very carefully strain the stock into a bowl and discard
the flavourings. Skim any fat from the surface and
use immediately, or leave it to cool completely. Once
cool it will be slightly gelled. See page 9 for storage
information.

TURKEY STOCK Prepare and store as Chicken Stock
but use broken turkey bones.

GAME STOCK Prepare and store as Chicken Stock but
use the bones from roast partridge, pheasant or other
game birds, reduce the water to 1.5l/52fl oz/6½ cups
and reduce the simmering time to 1½ hours. Makes
about 1.25l/44fl oz/5½ cups.

FISH STOCK

MAKES about 2l/70fl oz/2 quarts
PREPARATION TIME 10 minutes
COOKING TIME 30 minutes

1kg/2¼lb fish heads, bones and trimmings from white
    fish, such as hake, halibut, plaice/flounder or whiting,
    well rinsed to remove any blood and chopped
150ml/5fl oz/⅔ cup dry white wine
1 carrot, peeled and thinly sliced
1 large leek, thinly sliced and rinsed
1 onion, thinly sliced
1 bouquet garni made with several parsley sprigs and
    1 bay leaf tied together
½ lemon, thinly sliced
1 tsp black peppercorns, lightly crushed
a small pinch of salt

Put the fish heads, bones and trimmings in a large
saucepan. Add the wine and 2l/70fl oz/2 quarts
water, cover and bring to just below the boil, skimming
the surface as necessary. Add the remaining ingredients,
reduce the heat and simmer, covered, for 20 minutes.

Very carefully strain the stock into a bowl and discard the
flavourings. The stock is now ready to use. See page 9
for storage information.

VEGETABLE STOCK

MAKES about 2l/70fl oz/2 quarts
PREPARATION TIME 20 minutes
COOKING TIME 45 minutes

2 tbsp olive, hemp or sunflower oil
4 celery stalks, with the leaves, chopped
2 carrots, coarsely chopped
2 onions, finely chopped
1 leek, sliced and rinsed
6 garlic cloves
1 small tomato, chopped

1 bouquet garni made with 1 bay leaf and several
    parsley and thyme sprigs tied together
12 black peppercorns, lightly crushed
½ tsp salt
onion skins (optional)

Heat the oil in a saucepan over a medium heat. Stir in
the celery, carrots, onions and leek, then reduce the heat
to very low and cook, covered, for 10–15 minutes until
very soft. Add the remaining ingredients and 2.2l/77fl
oz/2¼ quarts water, then cover and bring to the
boil. Skim, then reduce the heat and simmer, partially
covered, for 20 minutes.

Very carefully strain the stock into a bowl and discard all
the flavourings. The stock is now ready to use. See page
9 for storage information.

DASHI

MAKES about 1.25l/44fl oz/5½ cups
PREPARATION TIME 5 minutes, plus 30 minutes
    soaking
COOKING TIME 20 minutes

25cm/10in piece of dried kombu
10g/¼oz/⅔ cup bonito (fish) flakes

Put the kombu and 1.4l/48fl oz/6 cups water in a
saucepan and leave to soak for 30 minutes.

Bring to the boil, uncovered. As soon as it boils, skim
the surface, then add the bonito flakes. Skim the surface
again, if necessary. Reduce the heat and simmer,
uncovered, for 10 minutes.

Strain the dashi into a large bowl and use immediately.
Alternatively, leave to cool, then store in the refrigerator
for up to 2 days. Freezing isn't recommended for more
than 2 weeks as it will lose much of its flavour.

VEGETARIAN DASHI Omit the bonito flakes in the
above recipe. Instead soak 8 dried shiitake mushrooms

in 1.4l/48fl oz/6 cups hot water for at least 30 minutes.
Put the mushrooms and the soaking liquid in a saucepan.
Add the kombu and leave to soak for 30 minutes. Slowly
bring to the boil, uncovered. As soon as it boils, skim the
surface, then reduce the heat and simmer, uncovered, for
10 minutes. Strain through a muslin-lined/cheesecloth-
lined sieve, and use the dashi as above.

INSTANT DASHI Many good-quality powdered dashi
mixes are sold in Japanese food shops, wholefood
shops and on the internet. Follow the instructions on
the package, which is usually to dissolve 2 teaspoons
powder in 1.25l/44fl oz/5½ cups water. If you are
a vegetarian, check the labelling closely, or ask an
assistant (it will be written in Japanese), because instant
dashi is made with and without bonito flakes.

BEEF CONSOMMÉ

MAKES 1.25l/44fl oz/5½ cups
PREPARATION TIME 15 minutes, plus 30 minutes
    chilling and slow straining
COOKING TIME 50 minutes

280g/10oz boneless shin of beef, minced/ground
1 carrot, peeled and diced
1 celery stalk, finely chopped
1 leek, thinly sliced and rinsed
3 egg whites
1 tbsp tomato purée/paste
1.5l/52fl oz/6½ cups Beef Stock (see page 11)
    or ready-made stock
salt and freshly ground black pepper

Mix the minced/ground beef, carrot, celery and leek
together in a large bowl. Beat the egg whites in another
bowl until frothy, then add the tomato purée/paste and
mix together. Add this mixture to the minced/ground
beef and stir together until well combined. Cover and
chill for 30 minutes.

Pour the stock into a saucepan, add the chilled egg-white mixture and season with salt and pepper. Slowly bring to the boil, stirring. As soon as the liquid is frothy, stop stirring. When the liquid comes to the boil, immediately reduce the heat to very low (use a heat diffuser if you have one) and simmer, without stirring, for 30–40 minutes until a solid crust forms.

Meanwhile, line a sieve with muslin/cheesecloth and set over a large bowl. Gently poke a hole in the centre of the crust to see if the stock is sparkling clear. When the stock is clear, increase the hole in the crust and use a ladle to transfer the stock through the muslin-lined/cheesecloth-lined sieve: do not push it through or squeeze the cloth. Once strained, the consommé is ready to use. Alternatively, leave to cool completely, cover and refrigerate for up to 2 days or freeze for up to 6 months.

CHICKEN CONSOMMÉ Make as above but replace the stock with Chicken Stock (see page 12) and the meat with very finely chopped or minced/ground boneless, skinless chicken legs.

ACCOMPANIMENTS

BIG WHITE LOAF

MAKES 1 large loaf
PREPARATION TIME 15 minutes, plus kneading, 3 risings and cooling
COOKING TIME 40 minutes

450g/1lb/3¼ cups strong white/white bread flour, plus extra for dusting
1½ tsp easy-blend/instant dried yeast
1 tsp sugar
2 tsp salt
30g/1oz/2 tbsp butter, at room temperature and diced
sunflower oil, for greasing
1 egg yolk, beaten, for glazing

The day before you plan to bake, put 150g/5½oz/heaped 1 cup of the flour, 1 teaspoon of the yeast and ½ teaspoon of the sugar in a mixing bowl. Slowly pour in 100ml/3½fl oz/7 tbsp water heated to 43°C/110°F and mix together. It will form a thick, sticky mixture. Cover the bowl with cling film/plastic wrap, then set aside for at least 8 hours, or until the mixture appears softer and has bubbles on the surface.

The next day, add the remaining flour, yeast, sugar and the salt, and stir together. Stir in the butter and make a well in the centre. Pour 175ml/6fl oz/¾ cup water heated to 43°C/110°F into the well and mix, gradually incorporating the flour from the side to make a soft, sticky dough. Slowly add up to 4 tablespoons extra water, if required, to make a soft dough.

Knead the dough in the bowl until a ball forms, then turn it out onto a lightly floured surface and knead for 10 minutes, or until it is elastic, no longer sticky and the butter has melted into the dough. Shape it into a ball.

Wash and dry the bowl and very lightly rub with oil. Put the dough ball in the bowl and roll it around so it is lightly coated with oil, then cover the bowl with cling film/plastic wrap and set aside in a warm place until the dough doubles in volume, which can take up to 2 hours. Meanwhile, heavily dust a baking sheet with extra flour. Punch down the dough, then turn it out onto a lightly floured surface and roll around for 1–2 minutes.

Pat the dough into a rectangle about 20 x 12cm/8 x 4½in. Fold the top edge down to the centre and press firmly. Fold the bottom edge up over the top, as if folding a letter, and press firmly. Turn the loaf over and roll it into a 25cm/10in oval shape with tapered ends. Place the loaf on the prepared baking sheet, cover with a dish towel and leave to rise until it doubles in volume. Meanwhile, preheat the oven to 220°C/425°F/Gas 7.

Very lightly brush the surface of the dough with the beaten egg: take care not to knock out any of the air.

Using a very sharp thin knife, make 2 shallow, long diagonal cuts on the surface.

Immediately put the bread in the oven and bake for 5 minutes. Reduce the heat to190°C/375°F/Gas 5 and bake for a further 30–35 minutes until the loaf is risen, golden brown and the bottom sounds hollow when tapped. Leave the loaf to cool completely on a wire/ cooling rack. This bread will keep fresh for 3 days in an airtight container, or can be frozen for up to 6 months.

BIG BROWN LOAF Make as above but replace half (or all) the white flour with strong wholemeal/ wholewheat bread flour.

WHOLEMEAL IRISH SODA BREAD

MAKES 1 loaf
PREPARATION TIME 10 minutes, plus cooling
COOKING TIME 40 minutes

450g/1lb/3¼ cups strong wholemeal/wholewheat
    bread flour, plus extra for dusting
2 tsp sugar
1 tsp baking powder
½ tsp salt
¼ tsp bicarbonate of soda/baking soda
55g/2oz/¼ cup butter, at room temperature and diced
300ml/10fl oz/1¼ cups buttermilk, plus extra, if needed
1 egg, beaten

Preheat the oven to 220°C/425°F/Gas 7 and heavily flour a baking sheet. Stir the flour, sugar, baking powder, salt and bicarbonate of soda/baking soda together. Rub in the butter until the mixture resembles fine breadcrumbs, then make a well in the centre.

Pour in the buttermilk, add the egg and mix together. Gradually stir in flour from the side and mix until a thick dough forms, adding a little extra buttermilk, if necessary.

Turn out onto a lightly floured surface and pat into a large ball. Place the dough ball on the prepared baking

sheet and make 2 diagonal cuts across the top with a very sharp thin knife, each about 2cm/¾in deep.

Put the baking sheet in the oven and bake for 10 minutes. Reduce the temperature to 200°C/400°F/Gas 6 and continue baking for 25–30 minutes until the bottom sounds hollow when tapped. Transfer the bread to a wire/cooling rack and leave to cool for 10–15 minutes, then wrap in a dish towel and leave to cool completely. This bread is best eaten on the day it is baked but it can be stored in an airtight container for up to a day, or can be frozen for up to 6 months.

WHITE IRISH SODA BREAD Make as above but replace the flour with strong white/white bread flour.

PULL-APARTS

MAKES 12
PREPARATION TIME 20 minutes, plus kneading,
    2 risings and cooling
COOKING TIME 35 minutes

225g/8oz/1⅔ cups strong white/white bread flour,
    plus extra for dusting
225g/8oz/1⅔ cups strong wholemeal/wholewheat
    bread flour
2 tbsp cornflour/cornstarch
1½ tbsp soft light brown sugar
1½ tsp easy-blend/instant dried yeast
1½ tsp salt
30g/1oz/2 tbsp butter, at room temperature and diced
150ml/5fl oz/⅔ cup milk
olive oil or hemp oil, for greasing the bowl and for
    brushing the rolls

Stir the flours, cornflour/cornstarch, sugar, yeast and salt together. Stir in the butter and make a well in the centre. Mix the milk with 125ml/4fl oz/½ cup water and heat to 43°C/110°F. Slowly pour the liquid into the well and mix, gradually incorporating the flour from the side to make a soft, sticky dough.

Knead the dough in the bowl until a ball forms, then turn it out onto a lightly floured surface and knead for 10 minutes, or until no longer sticky and the butter has melted into the dough. Shape it into a ball.

Wash and dry the bowl and very lightly rub with oil. Put the dough ball in the bowl and roll it around so it is lightly coated with oil, then cover the bowl with cling film/plastic wrap and set aside in a warm place until the dough doubles in volume, which can take up to 2 hours. Meanwhile, dust a baking sheet and set aside.

Punch down the dough, then turn it out onto a lightly floured surface and roll it around for 1–2 minutes. Cut the dough into 12 equal pieces and roll each piece of dough into a smooth ball. Arrange the balls on the prepared baking sheet in a rectangle shape of 3 rows with 4 balls each, gently pushed together and touching. Cover with a dish towel and leave to rise until the rolls double in volume, which depends on the room temperature. Meanwhile, preheat the oven to 180°C/350°F/Gas 4.

Put the rolls in the oven and bake for 30–35 minutes until risen and brown on top. Remove the baking sheet from the oven, place a dish towel over the rolls with a wire/cooling rack very gently on top of that. Wearing oven gloves, invert the baking sheet and wire/cooling rack, then tap the rolls on the bottom – if they sound hollow they are baked. If not, return them to the oven and bake for a further 5 minutes before re-testing. Transfer the rolls to a wire/cooling rack, brush with oil and leave to cool completely. These rolls will keep fresh for 3 days in an airtight container, or can be frozen for up to 6 months.

MINI PULL-APARTS (for children) – Make as above, but cut the dough into 24 equal pieces rather than 12. Bake for 20–25 minutes and test as above.

HERB GRISSINI

MAKES about 60
PREPARATION TIME 25 minutes, plus kneading,
    2 risings and cooling
COOKING TIME 20 minutes

350g/12oz/2½ cups strong white/white bread flour,
    plus extra for dusting
1 tbsp salt
¾ tsp easy-blend/instant dried yeast
a pinch of sugar
1 tbsp extra-virgin olive oil, plus extra for greasing
    and brushing
1 tbsp very finely chopped rosemary needles
½ tsp chopped marjoram leaves
freshly ground black pepper

Stir the flour, salt, yeast and sugar together. Make a well in the centre, add the olive oil and 175ml/6fl oz/ ¾ cup water heated to 43°C/110°F, holding back about 2 tablespoons of the water, and mix slowly. Gradually incorporate the flour from the side to make a soft dough.

Knead the dough in the bowl until a ball forms, then turn it out onto a lightly floured surface and knead for 10 minutes, or until it is elastic and no longer sticky, slowly adding the reserved liquid or a little extra flour, if necessary. Knead in the rosemary and marjoram.

Shape the dough into a ball. Wash and dry the bowl and very lightly rub with oil. Put the dough ball in the bowl and roll it around so it is lightly coated with oil. Cover the bowl with cling film/plastic wrap or a folded dish towel and set aside in a warm place until the dough doubles in volume, which can take up to 2 hours.

Brush two or three baking sheets with oil and set aside. Punch down the dough, then turn it out onto a lightly floured surface and knead it for 1–2 minutes. Cut the dough into 4 equal pieces. Lightly flour a rolling pin and roll a piece of dough until it is about 30cm/12in long and 5mm/¼in thick. Using a ruler and pizza cutter or a knife, cut out fifteen 5mm/¼in-wide strips.

Very lightly flour a work surface with a bit of texture, such as a wooden or plastic chopping board. Put a dough strip on the surface and roll it back and forth, stretching the height to around 30–38cm/12–15in. Place the grissini on one of the prepared baking sheets (about 5mm/¼in apart) and continue shaping the remaining grissini. Preheat the oven to 190°C/375°F/Gas 5, then brush the grissini with oil and cover lightly with a dish towel. Set aside to rise while the oven warms up. Baking in batches if necessary, bake for about 20 minutes, or until the grissini are crisp and golden brown. Gently transfer the grissini to a wire/cooling rack and leave to cool completely. Store for up to 3 days in an airtight container.

POLENTA DUMPLINGS

MAKES 12 or 24 dumplings
PREPARATION TIME 15 minutes
COOKING TIME 15 minutes

300g/10½oz/2 cups medium polenta
55g/2oz/scant ½ cup self-raising/self-rising flour, plus extra for shaping
½ tsp baking powder
3 tbsp finely chopped parsley or dill
¼ tsp salt
1 egg, beaten
3 tbsp milk
1 tbsp olive or hemp oil, plus extra if making the dumplings in advance

These can be shaped and cooked up to 1 day in advance. Mix the polenta, flour, baking powder, parsley and salt in a bowl. Make a well in the centre, add the egg, milk and oil, then gradually beat together until a thick, crumbly dough forms. Lightly flour your hands and divide the mixture into 12 or 24 equal pieces. Roll into

balls, taking care to smooth over all cracks and openings or the dumplings will become soggy. Meanwhile, bring a large saucepan of water to the boil. Reduce the heat so the water is just boiling. Add the dumplings and cook until they rise to the surface, then cook for another 10 minutes.

Use a slotted spoon to transfer the dumplings to the soup and finish as instructed in the recipe. If not using at once, transfer the dumplings to a plate and pour off any excess water. Leave to cool, then very lightly coat with oil to prevent them from sticking together, cover with cling film/plastic wrap and refrigerate for up to 1 day. Reheat in gently simmering soup.

CROÛTES

MAKES 4–6
PREPARATION TIME 5 minutes
COOKING TIME 6 minutes

4–6 slices of French bread, sliced on the diagonal
olive or hemp oil (optional)

Preheat the grill/broiler to high and position the grill/broiler rack 10cm/4in from the heat. Put the bread slices on the rack and toast for 2–3 minutes on each side until golden brown and crisp. Brush with oil, if desired, and serve warm or at room temperature. The croûtes can be stored in an airtight container for up to 3 days.

GARLIC CROÛTES Follow the recipe as above, but brush with garlic-flavoured oil.

GRUYÈRE OR CHEDDAR CROÛTES Follow the recipe as above. After brushing with oil, sprinkle with grated cheese and grill/broil until the cheese melts and is very lightly tinged. Serve warm.

GOATS' CHEESE CROÛTES Follow the recipe as above, but use a basil- or herb-flavoured olive oil, if you like. After brushing with oil, sprinkle with crumbled or chopped rindless goats' cheese and grill/broil until the cheese melts. Serve warm.

CROÛTONS

MAKES 4–6 servings
PREPARATION TIME 5 minutes
COOKING TIME 4–6 minutes

1 tbsp butter
olive or hemp oil
2 slices of day-old sliced white or wholemeal/wholewheat
    bread, cut into 0.5–1cm/¼–½in cubes, crusts removed

Croûtons are best made just before serving, so they are added to the soup hot. Line a plate with several layers of paper towels and set aside. Melt the butter with the oil in a large frying pan over a medium-high heat. Working in batches, if necessary, add the bread cubes and fry, stirring, for 2–3 minutes until golden brown and crisp.

Remove the croûtons from the pan and drain on the paper. If not using immediately, leave to cool completely, then store in an airtight container and reheat in a low oven before serving.

GARLIC CROÛTONS Follow the recipe as above, but use garlic-flavoured oil.

ROUILLE

MAKES about 175ml/6fl oz/¾ cup; enough for
    4–6 servings
PREPARATION TIME 10 minutes, plus chargrilling
    the pepper

55g/2oz/1 cup fresh breadcrumbs
2 large garlic cloves, chopped
1 large red pepper, chargrilled (see page 10), peeled,
    deseeded and chopped, or 1 roasted red pepper
    in oil, drained and chopped
125ml/4fl oz/½ cup extra-virgin olive oil, plus extra
    as needed
salt and cayenne pepper

Put the breadcrumbs, garlic and red pepper in a beaker or deep bowl and blend until a thick paste forms. Add half the olive oil, season with salt and cayenne and blend again. Slowly add the remaining oil, while blending, until a thick sauce forms. Cover and refrigerate for up to 2 days.

GREMOLATA

MAKES 4–6 servings
PREPARATION TIME 5 minutes

finely grated zest of 1 lemon
1 garlic clove, very finely chopped
3 tbsp finely chopped parsley leaves

Mix together all the ingredients in a bowl. (This is best made just before serving, although it will retain its fresh flavour for several hours, or overnight in the refrigerator.) Sprinkle gremolata over soups along with a drizzle of olive oil or other flavoured herb oil for a hit of fresh, zesty flavour.

FINISHING TOUCHES

Spiced Seeds – Heat a dry frying pan over a high heat. Add 30g/1oz/¼ cup each pumpkin and sunflower seeds, 3 tablespoons sesame seeds and 1 teaspoon fennel seeds, if desired, and cook, stirring, for 2–3 minutes until the seeds pop and start to colour. Immediately sprinkle over 1 tablespoon light soy sauce or tamari soy sauce and stir until evaporated. Transfer the seeds to a bowl and stir in ½ teaspoon celery seed. Store in an airtight container.

Roasted Pumpkin Seeds – Preheat the oven to 180°C/350°F/Gas 4. Dissolve ½ tablespoon salt in 500ml/18fl oz/2¼ cups water in a saucepan over a high heat. Add 75g/2¾oz/½ cup pumpkin seeds and bring to the boil. Immediately reduce the heat and simmer for 10 minutes. Drain and pat completely dry. Toss the seeds with 1 teaspoon olive or hemp oil and spread out on a baking sheet. Roast for 10–20 minutes, stirring frequently, until golden brown. Meanwhile, line a plate with several layers of paper towels. Transfer the seeds onto the paper and leave to cool. Store in a sealed container in the refrigerator for up to 2 weeks.

Chilli Bon-Bon – This piquant sherry is great for adding to curried soups as an alternative to hot pepper sauce. Fill a jar with medium or dry sherry and add 2 or 3 slit and deseeded bird's-eye chillies (plus extra, as desired). Seal the jar, shake and set aside for at least 5 days before using. This keeps indefinitely in the refrigerator or cupboard.

Crushed Herb Oils – Make this with basil, coriander/cilantro, mint or parsley leaves. Put a handful of leaves in a mortar with a pinch of salt and use a pestle to pound them to a paste. Slowly add olive or hemp oil, 1 tablespoon at a time, pounding until the oil is thick and fragrant. Adjust the salt and pepper, if necessary. These are best freshly made.

Chillies in Vinegar – This traditional accompaniment to Thai soups is usually made just before you start cooking the soup. Thickly slice long red chillies (not bird's-eye chillies unless you like very hot food), deseed if desired, and put them in a small bowl. Cover with distilled white vinegar and set aside until required.

Crisp-Fried Garlic – This is a traditional accompaniment to Thai soups that is usually prepared just before you start cooking the soup. Put 5 coarsely chopped garlic cloves in 5cm/2in olive, hemp or sunflower oil in a small saucepan over a high heat. Heat just until the garlic is golden brown and small bubbles appear around the edge, then immediately pour into a heatproof bowl and set aside to cool. Serve in little bowls for diners to add to their soup at the table, if they like.

Crisp-Fried Shallots – Cut 2 or 3 shallots in half lengthways, then thinly slice. Heat the oil and cook as above. If you remove the shallots and oil from the heat before they turn brown they will not over-cook in the residual heat and burn. When cool, use a slotted spoon to remove the shallots from the oil and drain on paper towels. Store in an airtight container for up to 2 days and use to sprinkle over soups.

Crunchy Mixed Seeds – Mix together 4 tablespoons each sunflower and pumpkin seeds, 2 tablespoons white sesame seeds, 1 tablespoon hemp seeds and 1 tablespoon lightly cracked flaxseed. Store covered in the refrigerator for up to 1 month.

Symbol key

Dairy-free

Nut-free (coconut is being treated as a nut in this book, so recipes with coconut milk have not been labelled as nut-free)

Wheat-free

V Vegetarian (no meat, game or seafood, but can contain dairy and egg products)

Vegan (no meat, game, seafood, dairy or egg products)

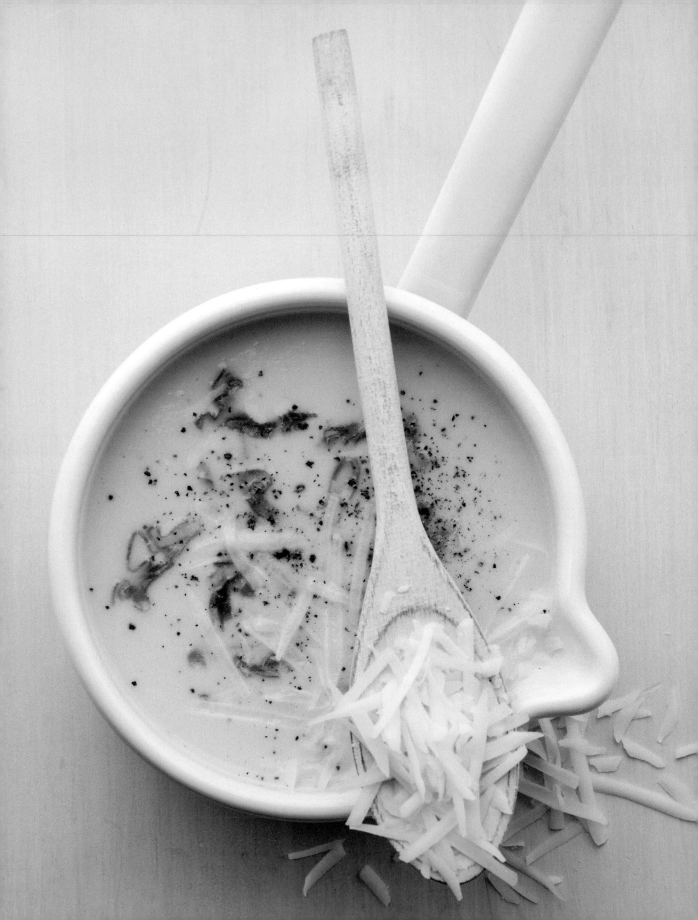

MEAT & GAME SOUPS

It's easy to think of meat soups as substantial winter meals, but light, spiced soups imbued with traditional flavours from Southeast Asia give this chapter a year-round appeal. Mrs Schultz's Beef & Vegetable Soup, for example, is a true winter warmer, but you will also find flavoursome lighter ideas, such as Thai Meatball & Coconut Soup.

Like most stews and casseroles, the slowly cooked meat soups in this chapter benefit from being made a day in advance. Borscht, Sausage, Fennel & Bean Soup and Syrian Red Lentil & Lamb Soup are examples of filling main-course soups that are best made ahead for quick reheating at mealtime. They are perfect for family meals after a busy workday or when you are casually entertaining.

Rich meat soups can be surprisingly economical, too. Portuguese Caldo Verde, Split Pea & Ham Soup and Scotch Broth make filling soups that don't cost a lot to make, but are certain to please.

MRS SCHULTZ'S BEEF
& VEGETABLE SOUP

PREPARATION TIME 15 minutes, plus making the stock

COOKING TIME 2 hours

2 tbsp garlic-flavoured sunflower oil,
plus extra as needed

450g/1lb stewing steak, cut into bite-size pieces
and patted dry

1 onion, finely chopped

¼ tsp paprika

125ml/4fl oz/½ cup dry red wine

750ml/26fl oz/3¼ cups Beef Stock (see page
11) or ready-made stock

1 can (400g/14oz) chopped tomatoes

2 bay leaves

1 carrot, peeled, halved lengthways and
thickly sliced

1 floury/russet potato, peeled and diced

½ celery stalk, finely chopped

salt and freshly ground black pepper

chopped parsley leaves, to serve

Heat 1½ tablespoons of the oil in a saucepan over a medium-high heat. Working in batches, if necessary, to avoid overcrowding the pan, fry the beef for 2–3 minutes until browned on all sides, then transfer to a plate and set aside. Add more oil between batches, if necessary.

Add the remaining oil to the pan and heat. Add the onion and fry, stirring occasionally, for 3–5 minutes until softened but not coloured. Return the beef and any accumulated juices to the pan, and add the paprika. Stir in the wine and cook for 5–6 minutes until almost evaporated.

Add the stock, then cover and bring to the boil. Skim the surface, then add the tomatoes and bay leaves and season with salt and pepper. Cover and return to the boil, then reduce the heat to very low (use a heat diffuser if you have one) and simmer for 1 hour.

Stir in the carrot, potato and celery and simmer, covered, for 30–45 minutes until the beef and vegetables are tender. Discard the bay leaves, then adjust the salt and pepper, if necessary. Serve immediately, sprinkled with parsley.

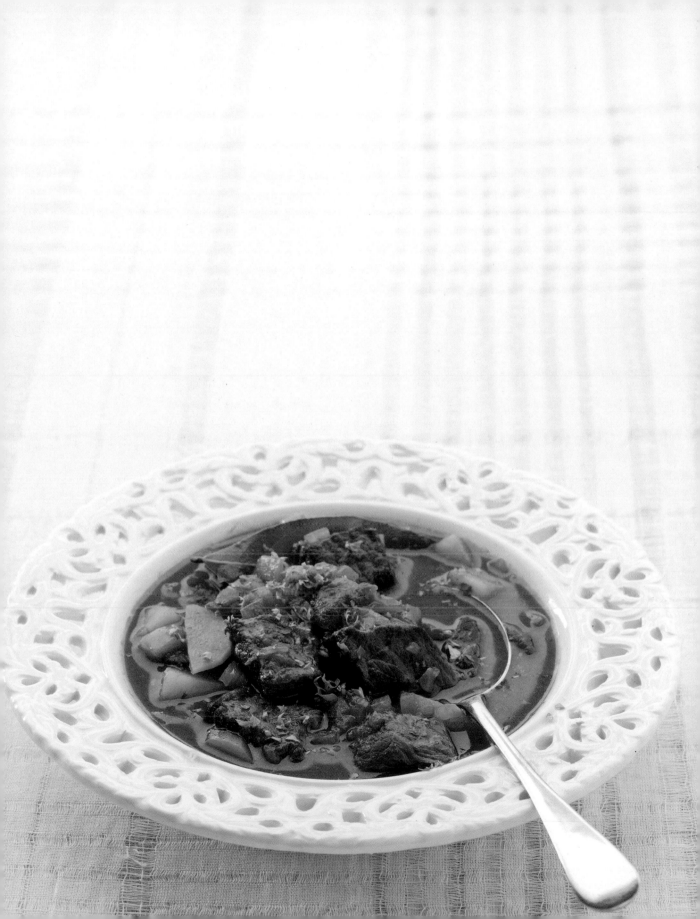

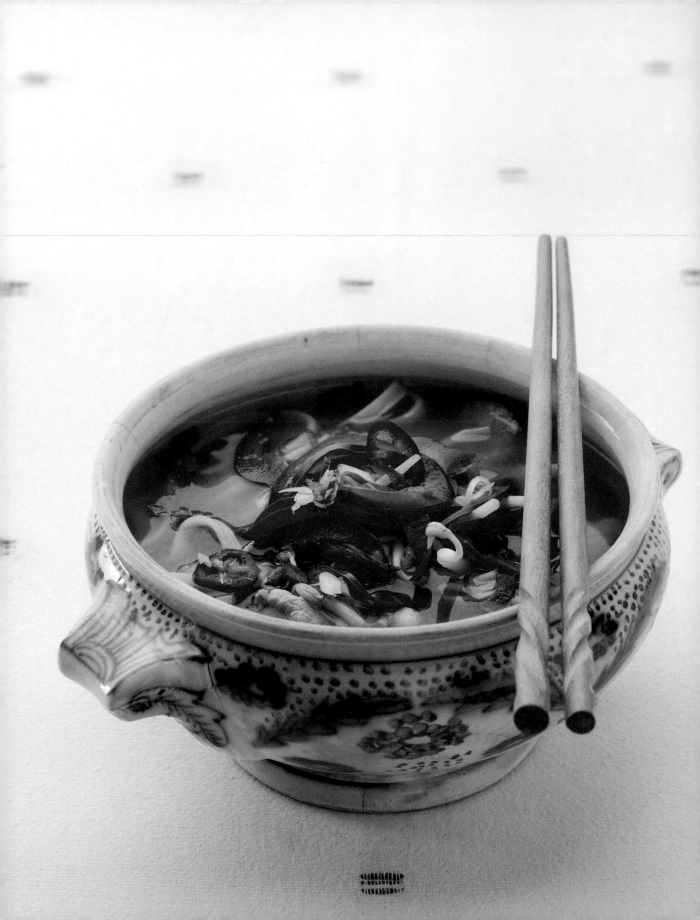

VIETNAMESE BEEF & NOODLE SOUP

PREPARATION TIME 20 minutes, plus making the stock

COOKING TIME 20 minutes

1 small handful of bean sprouts

1.75l/60fl oz/7½ cups Beef Stock (see page 11)

4cm/1½in piece of fresh ginger, peeled and thinly sliced

4 star anise

1 cinnamon stick

seeds from 4 green cardamom pods

1 tbsp fish sauce, or to taste

1 red pepper, halved, deseeded and very thinly sliced

500g/1lb 2oz medium-width ready-to-eat rice noodles

600g/1lb 5oz beef sirloin, rump or topside, in one piece, very thinly sliced against the grain

TO SERVE

lime wedges

1 handful of mint leaves

1 handful of coriander/cilantro leaves

2 spring onions/scallions, thinly sliced

thinly sliced red chillies

Put the bean sprouts in a bowl, cover with cold water and set aside. Put the stock, ginger, star anise, cinnamon stick, cardamom seeds and fish sauce in a large saucepan. Cover and bring to the boil, then reduce the heat and simmer for 10 minutes. Add the red pepper slices for the final 3 minutes of simmering to soften them.

Just before serving, use a slotted spoon to scoop the spices out of the stock and discard, then return the stock to the boil. Put the noodles in a heatproof bowl, cover with boiling water and leave to soak for 15–30 seconds to warm through. Drain and divide into serving bowls, then divide the beef into the bowls.

Drain the bean sprouts and add them to the bowls. Ladle the boiling stock and red peppers over and serve immediately with lime wedges and small bowls of mint, coriander/cilantro, spring onions/scallions and chillies on the side.

ITALIAN WEDDING SOUP

PREPARATION TIME 35 minutes, plus making the stock and 30 minutes chilling
COOKING TIME 1¼ hours

1.75l/60fl oz/7½ cups Beef Stock (see page 11) or ready-made stock

1 Parmesan cheese rind, about 7.5 x 5cm/ 3 x 2in (see page 9)

1 Parma ham/prosciutto heel (see page 9)

1 bay leaf

2 tbsp fruity extra-virgin olive oil, plus extra to serve

2 celery stalks, finely chopped

1 onion, finely chopped

2 garlic cloves, chopped

250g/9oz/3½ cups escarole or curly kale leaves, chopped

100g/3½oz/1½ cups chopped spinach

salt and freshly ground black pepper

freshly grated Parmesan cheese, to serve

VEAL MEATBALLS
55g/2oz/½ cup dried breadcrumbs

4 tbsp milk

800g/1¾lb minced/ground veal

5 garlic cloves, finely chopped

4 spring onions/scallions, very finely chopped

3 tbsp very finely chopped parsley leaves

3 tbsp very finely chopped dill

85g/3oz/¾ cup finely grated Parmesan cheese

2 eggs, beaten

olive oil, for frying

The meatballs can be made up to 1 day in advance. Put the breadcrumbs and milk in a bowl and leave to soak. Meanwhile, line a baking sheet or two plates that will fit in your refrigerator with greaseproof/wax paper. Put the veal, garlic, spring onions/scallions, parsley, dill and cheese in a large bowl, add the breadcrumb mixture and season with salt and pepper. Add the egg little by little and work it into the mixture with your fingers. Fry a small amount of the mixture to test for seasoning.

With wet hands, divide the mixture into 12 equal portions, then divide each portion into 6 equal portions to make a total of 72. Roll into meatballs and put them on the baking sheet. Cover with cling film/plastic wrap and chill for at least 30 minutes.

Meanwhile, put the stock, cheese rind, ham heel and bay leaf in a saucepan. Cover and bring to the boil, then reduce the heat to very low (use a heat diffuser if you have one) and simmer while you fry the meatballs.

To fry the meatballs, heat one or two large frying pans over a high heat until a splash of water 'dances' on the surface. Add a thin layer of olive oil, reduce the heat to medium and add as many meatballs as will fit without overcrowding the pan. Fry the meatballs, turning gently, for 5–8 minutes until golden brown. Drain on paper towels and set aside until required. (At this point they can be left to cool completely and chilled for up to 24 hours.)

To finish making the soup, heat the olive oil in another large saucepan over a medium heat. Stir in the celery, onion and garlic, reduce the heat to low and cook, covered, for 10–12 minutes until softened but not coloured. Add the stock, along with the cheese rind, ham heel and bay leaf, cover and bring to the boil. Add the escarole and spinach, reduce the heat and simmer, covered, for 30 minutes.

Gently add the meatballs and simmer for another 5 minutes until warmed through. Season with salt and pepper, but remember the cheese rind and ham heel will have been salty.

Discard the cheese rind, ham heel and bay leaf. Divide the meatballs and greens into bowls and ladle the soup over them. Serve immediately with olive oil and grated Parmesan cheese on the side.

BEEF CONSOMMÉ WITH PORCINI MUSHROOMS

PREPARATION TIME 15 minutes, plus making
   the consommé and 30 minutes soaking
   the mushrooms
COOKING TIME 5 minutes

30g/1oz dried porcini mushrooms
1.25l/44fl oz/5½ cups Beef Consommé
   (see page 13)
1 tbsp dry sherry (optional)
salt (optional)
chopped parsley leaves, to serve

Put the mushrooms in a heatproof bowl, cover with boiling water and leave to soak for 30 minutes until tender. Strain through a muslin-lined/cheesecloth-lined sieve. (The soaking liquid can be used in another recipe or frozen until required.) Squeeze the mushrooms, trim the bases of the stalks/stems, if necessary, then thinly slice the caps and stalks and divide them into serving bowls.

Put the consommé in a saucepan over a high heat and heat to just below the boil. Stir in the sherry, if using, and season with salt, if required. Ladle the consommé over the mushrooms, sprinkle with parsley and serve immediately.

BORSCHT

PREPARATION TIME 25 minutes, plus making the stock and horseradish cream

COOKING TIME 2½ hours

1kg/2¼lb boneless beef silverside, brisket or chuck, in one piece

1.75l/60fl oz/7½ cups Beef Stock (see page 11) or ready-made stock

4 carrots, peeled and sliced

4 large tomatoes, coarsely chopped

3 celery stalks, sliced, with the leaves reserved

2 onions, halved and studded with several cloves in each half

2 tbsp tomato purée/paste

1 bouquet garni made with the celery leaves, 2 bay leaves, a small handful of parsley sprigs and several dill sprigs tied together

a pinch of sugar

4 large cooked beetroots/beets, peeled and coarsely grated

2 bay leaves

2 tbsp red wine vinegar

salt and freshly ground black pepper

1 recipe quantity Horseradish & Dill Cream (see page 154), to serve

chopped dill, to serve

Put the beef, stock, carrots, tomatoes, celery, onions, tomato purée/paste, bouquet garni and sugar in a saucepan and season with salt and pepper. Cover and bring to the boil. Skim, then reduce the heat to very low (use a heat diffuser if you have one) and simmer, covered, for 2 hours until the meat is tender.

Remove the beef from the pan and set aside until cool enough to handle. Strain the soup, pressing down to extract as much flavour as possible, then discard the flavourings and return the stock to the pan.

Remove any sinew from the beef, cut the meat into bite-size pieces and return it to the soup. Add the beetroots/beets, bay leaves and vinegar and simmer, covered, for 15 minutes until the beef is very tender. Discard the bay leaves and adjust the salt and pepper, if necessary. Serve topped with the horseradish cream and sprinkled with dill.

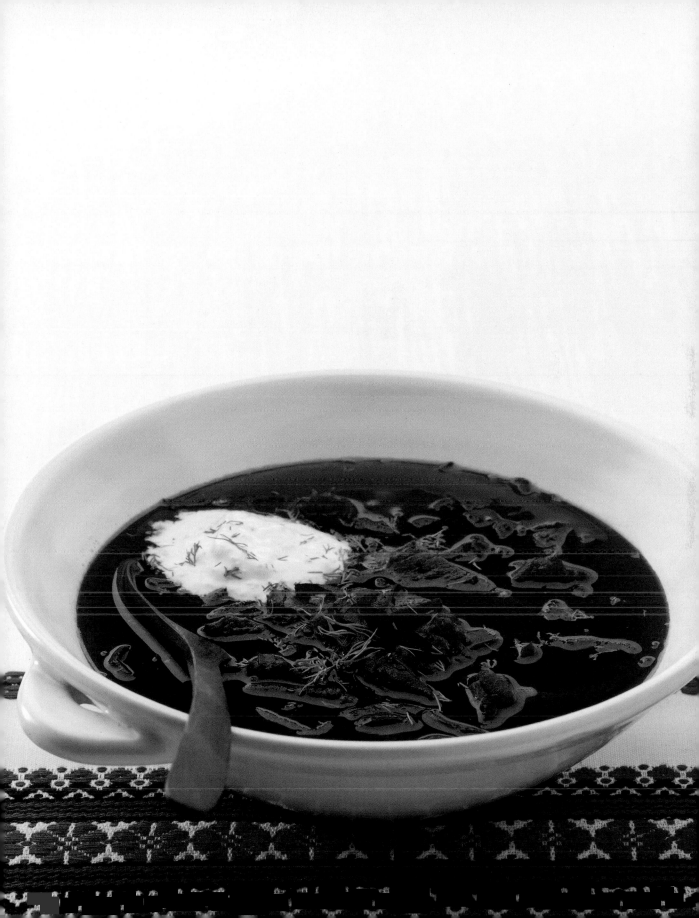

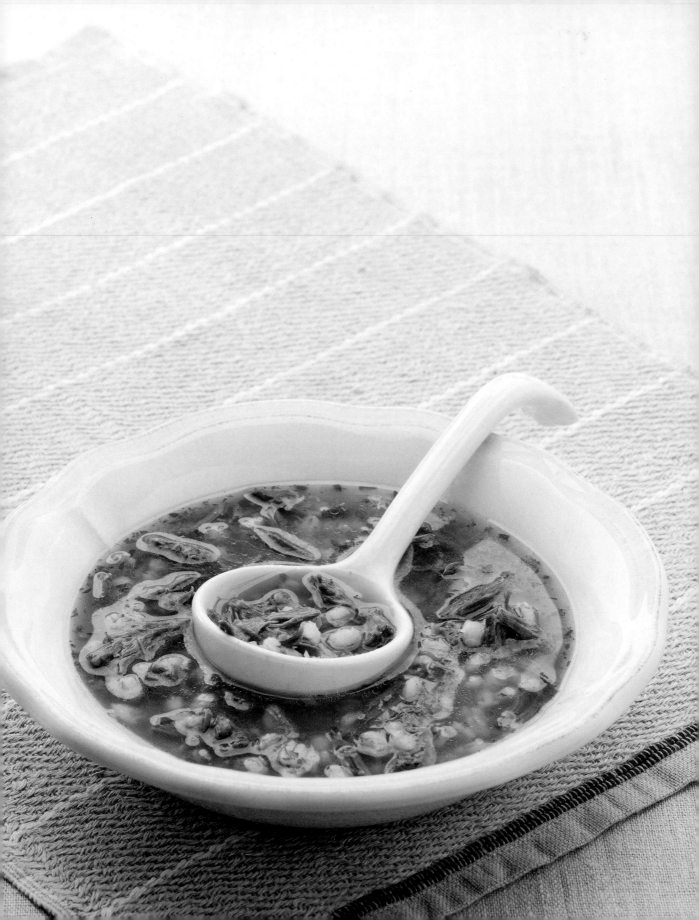

OXTAIL SOUP WITH BARLEY

PREPARATION TIME 20 minutes, plus overnight chilling (optional)

COOKING TIME 4 hours

2 tbsp butter

2 tbsp sunflower or olive oil, plus extra as needed

1kg/2¼lb oxtail, cut into large pieces (ask the butcher to do this)

3 celery stalks, chopped, with the leaves reserved

2 carrots, peeled and chopped

2 onions, chopped

4 garlic cloves, finely chopped

1 bouquet garni made with the reserved celery leaves, 1 bay leaf and several parsley and thyme sprigs tied together

85g/3oz/⅓ cup pearl barley

Worcestershire sauce, to taste

4 tbsp finely chopped parsley leaves

salt and freshly ground black pepper

This soup is best made a day before serving. Melt the butter with the oil in a large saucepan over a medium heat. Working in batches, fry the oxtail for 2–3 minutes until browned on both sides (add more oil if necessary), then transfer it to a plate.

Pour off all but 1½ tablespoons of the fat from the pan. Add the celery, carrots and onions and fry, stirring, for 2 minutes. Add the garlic and fry for 1–3 minutes until the onions are softened. Return the oxtail and any juices to the pan, add 2.5l/88fl oz/2½ quarts water and season with salt and pepper. Cover and bring to the boil, then skim and add the bouquet garni. Reduce the heat and simmer, covered, for 2½–3 hours until the meat is falling off the bones. Remove the meat and bones from the pan and set aside until cool enough to handle. Strain the soup into a clean pan, discarding the vegetables, and skim. Alternatively, leave the soup to cool completely, then cover and chill overnight for easier removal of the fat. (Spoon a little of the soup over the meat, before covering and chilling until required.)

Add the barley, cover and bring to the boil. Reduce the heat and simmer for 30–40 minutes until tender. Meanwhile, remove any skin and all the gristle from the meat and discard, along with the bones. Shred the meat, return it to the pan and reheat. Stir in the Worcestershire sauce and parsley. Adjust the salt and pepper, if necessary, and serve.

OSSO BUCO SOUP WITH GREMOLATA

PREPARATION TIME 15 minutes, plus making the stock and gremolata
COOKING TIME 2 hours

2–3 tbsp olive oil, plus extra as needed

600g/1lb 5oz bone-in osso buco or veal shin, about 3 thick pieces

2 shallots, finely chopped

1 carrot, peeled and diced

1 celery stalk, thinly chopped

4 large garlic cloves, very finely chopped

1.5l/52fl oz/6½ cups Beef Stock (see page 11) or ready-made stock

125ml/4fl oz/½ cup dry vermouth

500ml/18fl oz/2¼ cups passata (Italian sieved tomatoes)

1 bay leaf

1 tbsp tomato purée/paste

½ tsp sugar

a pinch of saffron threads

salt and freshly ground black pepper

1 recipe quantity Gremolata (see page 18), to serve

Heat 2 tablespoons of the oil in a saucepan over a medium heat. Working in batches, if necessary, to avoid overcrowding the pan, fry the osso buco for 2–3 minutes, turning occasionally, until browned on all sides. Remove from the pan and set aside. Add more oil between batches, if necessary.

Add the shallots, carrot and celery and fry, stirring occasionally, for 2 minutes. Add the garlic and fry for 1–3 minutes until the onion is softened but not coloured. Return the meat and any accumulated juices to the pan, add the stock and vermouth and season with salt and pepper. Cover and bring to the boil.

Skim, then add the passata, bay leaf, tomato purée/paste, sugar and saffron and season again with salt and pepper. Reduce the heat to very low (use a heat diffuser if you have one) and simmer, covered, for 1½–1¾ hours until the meat is very tender. Remove the meat from the soup and set aside until cool enough to handle.

Remove the meat from the bones, finely shred it and return it to the soup. Use a small spoon or knife to push the marrow out of the middle of the bones and stir it into the soup, if you like. Adjust the salt and pepper, if necessary, then skim. Serve sprinkled with the gremolata.

WINTER LAMB & ONION SOUP

PREPARATION TIME 10 minutes, plus making the stock

COOKING TIME 55 minutes

3 tbsp olive or hemp oil

400g/14oz boneless lamb neck fillet/tenderloin, membrane removed and meat patted dry

4 large onions, thinly sliced

1 tsp dried mint leaves

½ tsp ground cumin

½ tsp fenugreek seeds, lightly crushed

½ tsp turmeric

2 tbsp plain white/all-purpose or wholemeal/wholewheat flour

1l/35fl oz/4½ cups Chicken Stock (see page 12) or ready-made stock

1 cinnamon stick, broken in half

2 tbsp lemon juice

1 tsp sugar

salt and freshly ground black pepper

1 small handful of coriander/cilantro leaves, to serve

Heat 2 tablespoons of the oil in a saucepan over a medium heat. Add the lamb and fry, turning often, for 4 minutes until browned all over. Remove from the pan and set aside.

Add the remaining oil to the pan and heat. Add the onions and season with salt and pepper. Reduce the heat to low and cook, covered, for 10–12 minutes, stirring occasionally, until very soft and just starting to colour. Add the mint, cumin, fenugreek seeds and turmeric and stir for 30 seconds. Sprinkle in the flour and cook, stirring, for another 2 minutes. Remove the pan from the heat and slowly pour in the stock, stirring continuously, then add the cinnamon stick.

Bring to the boil, then reduce the heat to very low and simmer, partially covered, for 15 minutes. Meanwhile, cut the lamb across the grain into very thin slices, then cut any large slices in half.

Add the lamb to the soup and simmer for another 10 minutes or until the lamb is cooked to your liking. Discard the cinnamon stick and stir in the lemon juice and sugar. Adjust the salt and pepper, if necessary, then serve sprinkled with the coriander/cilantro.

SYRIAN RED LENTIL & LAMB SOUP

PREPARATION TIME 10 minutes, plus making the stock

COOKING TIME 1¼ hours

1.25l/44fl oz/5½ cups Vegetable Stock (see page 12) or water

650g/1½lb lamb shoulder chops

250g/9oz/1¼ cups split red lentils, rinsed and picked over

1 carrot, peeled and chopped

1 onion, finely chopped

1 tsp dried mint leaves

½ tsp ground coriander

½ tsp ground cumin

½ tsp chilli powder

a pinch of saffron threads

salt and freshly ground black pepper

chopped coriander/cilantro or parsley leaves, to serve

lemon wedges, to serve

hot pepper sauce, to serve (optional)

Put the stock, lamb, lentils, carrot, onion, mint, ground coriander, cumin, chilli powder and saffron in a saucepan. Cover and bring to the boil. Reduce the heat to very low (use a heat diffuser if you have one) and simmer for 1–1¼ hours until the lamb is tender and the lentils have fallen apart.

Remove the lamb and bones from the soup and set aside until cool enough to handle. Skim the soup, if necessary. Cut the meat from the bones into bite-size pieces and return it to the soup. Stir well and season with salt and pepper.

Serve sprinkled with coriander/cilantro leaves and with lemon wedges for squeezing over and hot pepper sauce for adding at the table, if you like.

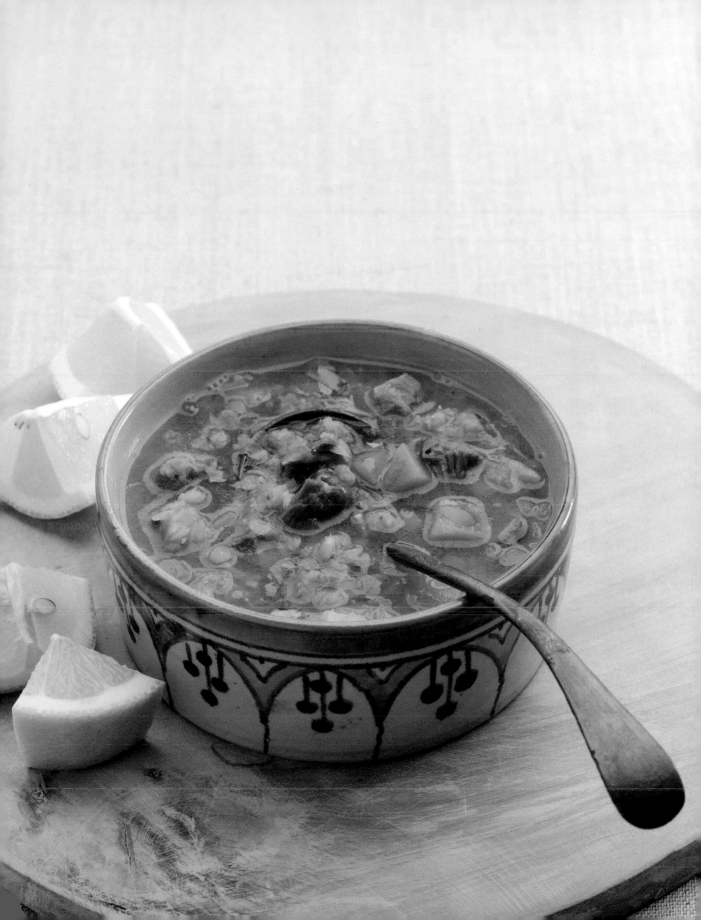

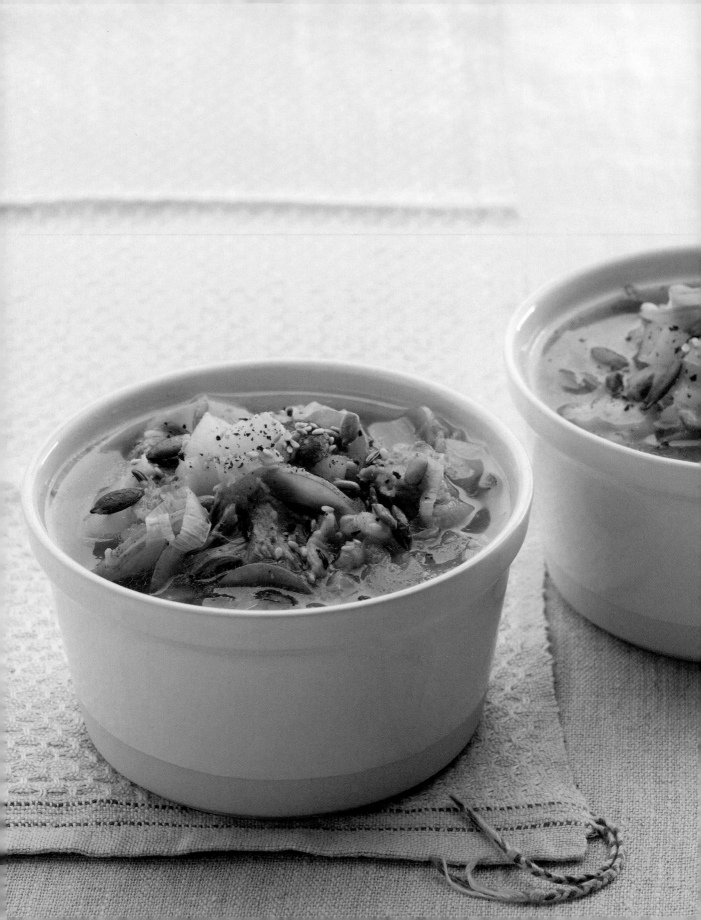

WELSH MOUNTAIN LAMB
& LEEK SOUP

PREPARATION TIME 20 minutes, plus making the seeds

COOKING TIME 1¾ hours

600g/1lb 5oz boneless shoulder of lamb, in one piece, trimmed

4 large garlic cloves, crushed

3 carrots, 2 coarsely chopped and 1 sliced

3 celery stalks

3 large leeks, 2 thickly sliced and 1 thinly sliced, all rinsed and kept separate

1 bouquet garni made with 2 bay leaves and several parsley and rosemary sprigs tied together

350g/12oz floury/russet potatoes, peeled and chopped

salt and freshly ground black pepper

Spiced Seeds (see page 19), to serve

Put the lamb and 1.25l/44fl oz/5½ cups water in a saucepan. Cover and bring to the boil. Skim, then add the garlic, chopped carrots, celery, thickly sliced leeks and bouquet garni. Season with salt and pepper, then reduce the heat and simmer, covered, for 1 hour.

Strain the stock and discard the vegetables and bouquet garni. Return the lamb and stock to the pan, then skim the fat from the surface. Add the sliced carrots, thinly sliced leeks and potatoes. Cover and bring to the boil, then reduce the heat and simmer for 30–45 minutes until the meat is meltingly tender and the potatoes are falling apart. Skim again, if necessary, then remove the lamb and set aside until cool enough to handle.

Cut the lamb into bite-size pieces, return it to the soup and reheat. Adjust the salt and pepper, if necessary, and serve sprinkled with the seeds.

ROAST LAMB & BEAN SOUP

PREPARATION TIME 15 minutes, plus making the stock and roasting the lamb

COOKING TIME 40 minutes

1 tbsp olive or hemp oil

1 red onion, finely chopped

3 garlic cloves, finely chopped

1 tsp ground coriander

½ tsp ground cumin

½ tsp turmeric

1l/35fl oz/4½ cups Beef Stock (see page 11) or ready-made stock

1 can (400g/14oz) chopped tomatoes

1 tbsp tomato purée/paste

½ tbsp dried mint leaves or dill

1 tsp harissa, or to taste

½ tsp sugar

1 lamb bone, all fat removed (optional)

400g/14oz boneless, skinless roast lamb, shredded with all fat removed

1 can (400g/14oz) cannellini beans or chickpeas/garbanzo beans, drained and rinsed

salt and freshly ground black pepper

chopped coriander/cilantro leaves, to serve

Heat the oil in a saucepan over a medium heat. Add the onion and fry, stirring occasionally, for 2 minutes. Add the garlic and fry for 1–3 minutes until the onion is softened but not coloured. Add the ground coriander, cumin and turmeric and stir for 30 seconds until aromatic. Watch closely so the spices do not burn.

Add the stock, tomatoes, tomato purée/paste, mint, harissa, sugar and lamb bone, if using. Season with salt and pepper, cover and bring to the boil over a high heat. Reduce the heat and simmer for 20 minutes, stirring once or twice to break up the tomatoes. Add the lamb and beans and simmer for 5 minutes to heat through. Discard the lamb bone, if used, then adjust the salt and pepper, if necessary, and add more harissa, if you like. Serve sprinkled with coriander/cilantro leaves.

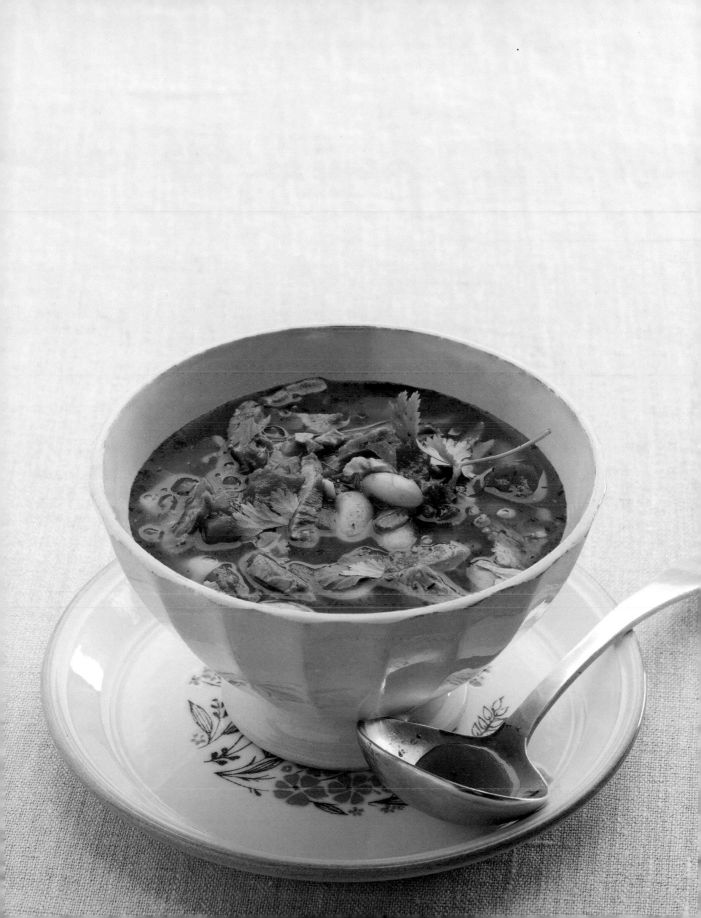

SCOTCH BROTH

PREPARATION TIME 15 minutes

COOKING TIME 1¾ hours

1kg/2¼lb neck of lamb on the bone, trimmed and chopped into pieces (ask the butcher to do this)

1 bouquet garni made with 1 piece of celery stalk, 1 bay leaf and several parsley and thyme sprigs tied together

55g/2oz/¼ cup pearl barley

2 leeks, thinly sliced and rinsed

1 carrot, peeled and diced

1 onion, finely chopped

1 turnip, peeled and diced

2 tbsp chopped parsley leaves

salt and freshly ground black pepper

Put the lamb and 1.75l/60fl oz/7½ cups water in a saucepan. Cover and slowly bring to just below the boil. Skim, then add the bouquet garni. Reduce the heat and simmer, covered, for 1 hour.

Stir in the barley, leeks, carrot, onion and turnip and return to just below the boil. Reduce the heat and simmer, covered, for 30–40 minutes until the meat and barley are tender. Remove the meat from the soup and set aside until cool enough to handle. Discard the bouquet garni.

Pull the meat away from the bones, cut it into small pieces and return it to the soup. Reheat, if necessary, then stir in the parsley. Season with salt and pepper and serve.

HAM & CHEESE CHICORY SOUP

PREPARATION TIME 15 minutes, plus making the stock

COOKING TIME 30 minutes

2 tbsp butter

1 tbsp olive oil

leaves from 4 heads of chicory/Belgian endive, coarsely chopped

1 floury/russet potato, peeled and diced

600ml/20fl oz/2½ cups Vegetable Stock (see page 12) or ready-made stock

1 Parmesan cheese rind, about 7.5 x 5cm/ 3 x 2in (see page 9; optional)

5 tbsp double/heavy cream

salt and ground white pepper

40g/1½oz thinly sliced Parma ham/prosciutto, to serve

freshly grated Gruyère cheese, to serve

Melt the butter with the oil in a saucepan over a medium heat. Add the chicory/endive and potato and fry, stirring, for 3–5 minutes until the chicory/ endive wilts but does not brown. Add the stock, 600ml/20fl oz/2½ cups water and the cheese rind, if using.

Cover and bring to the boil, then reduce the heat and simmer for 10–12 minutes until the potato is very tender. Discard the cheese rind, if used, add the cream and blend the soup until smooth. Season with salt and white pepper, and serve sprinkled with the ham and grated cheese.

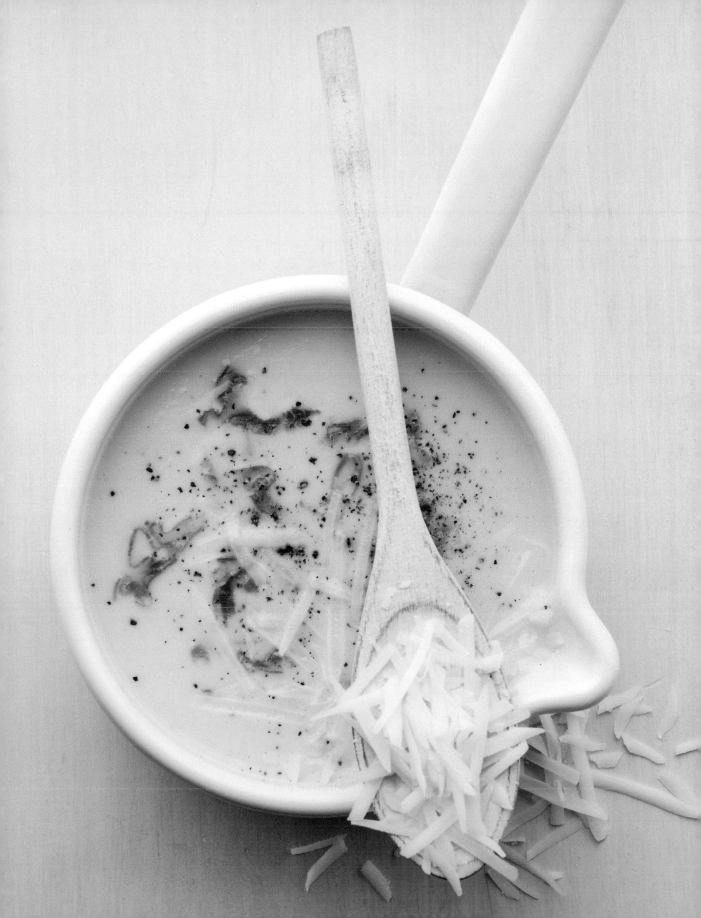

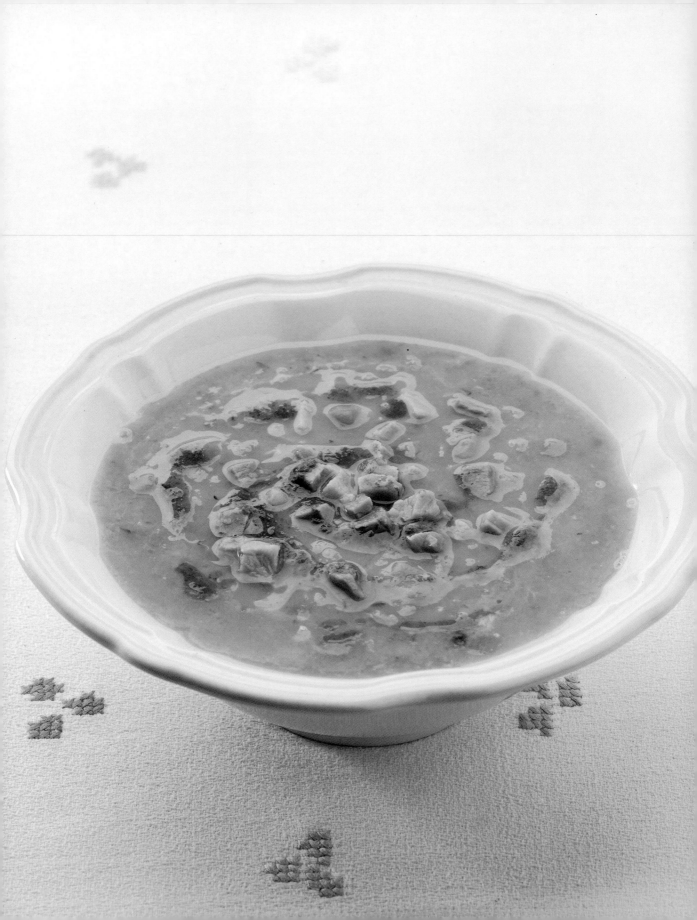

SPLIT PEA & HAM SOUP

PREPARATION TIME 15 minutes, plus making the flavoured oil

COOKING TIME 2¼ hours

2 tbsp sunflower oil

2 celery stalks, finely chopped

1 carrot, peeled and finely chopped

1 onion, finely chopped

1 cooked unsmoked gammon/ham bone with any meat that is left on it

200g/7oz/1 cup green split peas, rinsed

2 bay leaves

½ tbsp dried thyme leaves

350g/12oz/2 cups shredded or finely diced cooked ham

sugar, to taste (optional)

salt and freshly ground black pepper

1 recipe quantity Crushed Mint Oil (see page 19), to serve

Heat the oil in a large saucepan over a medium heat. Stir in the celery, carrot and onion, then reduce the heat to low, cover and cook, stirring occasionally, for 8–10 minutes until softened but not coloured.

Add the gammon/ham bone and split peas to the pan and stir in 1.6l/56fl oz/7 cups water. Cover and bring to the boil. Skim, if necessary. Stir in the bay leaves and thyme, reduce the heat to very low (use a heat diffuser if you have one) and simmer, covered, for 1½–2 hours, stirring frequently until the split peas are very tender and have thickened the soup and any meat is coming away from the bone.

Remove the bone from the pan and set aside. When it is cool enough to handle, shred any meat that might have been on it. Return the meat to the soup, add the cooked ham and reheat. Adjust the salt and pepper, if necessary, but remember the gammon/ham bone will have been salty so you might only need pepper; if the soup is too salty, stir in a little sugar. Serve drizzled with the mint oil.

SMOKED HAM & CELERY CHOWDER

PREPARATION TIME 20 minutes, plus making the stock

COOKING TIME 35 minutes

1 tbsp butter

1½ tbsp sunflower oil

400g/14oz/3 cups diced lean smoked ham, rind and any fat removed

2 celery stalks, finely chopped, with the leaves reserved to serve

1 leek, halved lengthways, sliced and rinsed

1 large floury/russet potato, peeled and diced

2 tbsp plain white/all-purpose or wholemeal/ wholewheat flour

500ml/18fl oz/2¼ cups Chicken Stock (see page 12) or ready-made stock

700ml/24fl oz/3 cups milk

2 tbsp chopped parsley leaves

1 bay leaf

finely grated zest of 1 lemon

4 tbsp sour cream

celery salt

freshly ground black pepper

celery seeds, to serve

Melt the butter with 1 tablespoon of the oil in a saucepan over a medium heat. Add the ham and fry, stirring, for 2–3 minutes until just starting to crisp on the edges. Remove it from the pan and set aside.

Add the remaining oil to the pan. Add the celery and leek and fry, stirring occasionally, for 3–5 minutes until the leek is softened but not coloured. Stir in the potato and return the ham to the pan, then sprinkle in the flour and stir for 2 minutes. Slowly add half the stock, scraping the base of the pan and stirring continuously to prevent lumps from forming.

Stir in the remaining stock, cover and bring to the boil, then skim. Reduce the heat to low and stir in the milk, parsley, bay leaf and lemon zest. Simmer, covered, for 15–18 minutes until the potato is starting to fall apart. Do not allow the soup to boil. Meanwhile, finely shred the reserved celery leaves.

Discard the bay leaf, stir in the sour cream and warm through. Season with celery salt and pepper, but remember the ham is salty. Serve sprinkled with celery leaves and seeds.

SAUSAGE, FENNEL & BEAN SOUP

PREPARATION TIME 15 minutes, plus overnight soaking
and cooking the beans (optional) and making the stock

COOKING TIME 30 minutes

200g/7oz/1 cup dried cannellini beans or
1 can (400g/14oz) cannellini beans, drained
and rinsed

1½ tbsp garlic-flavoured olive oil

400g/14oz spicy Italian sausages,
casings removed

1 celery stalk, finely chopped

1 fennel bulb, thinly sliced

1.25l/44fl oz/5½ cups Beef Stock (see page 11)
or ready-made stock

2 carrots, peeled and diced

2 bay leaves

salt and freshly ground black pepper

chopped parsley leaves, to serve

If using dried beans, put them in a bowl, cover with water and leave to soak overnight, then drain. Transfer to a saucepan, add 1.5l/52fl oz/6½ cups water, cover and bring to the boil. Reduce the heat and simmer, covered, for 50 minutes–1 hour until tender, then drain.

Heat the oil in a saucepan over a medium heat. Add the sausage meat and fry for 2–3 minutes, breaking up the meat, until browned all over. Remove the meat from the pan and set aside to drain on paper towels. Spoon off all but 1 tablespoon of the oil remaining in the pan. Add the celery and fennel and fry, stirring occasionally, for 8–10 minutes until light golden brown. Add the stock, carrots and bay leaves and season with salt and pepper.

Cover and bring to the boil. Skim, if necessary, then reduce the heat and simmer for 5 minutes. Return the sausage meat to the pan, add the beans and simmer for 2–3 minutes to warm through. Discard the bay leaves and skim again. Adjust the salt and pepper, if necessary, then serve sprinkled with parsley.

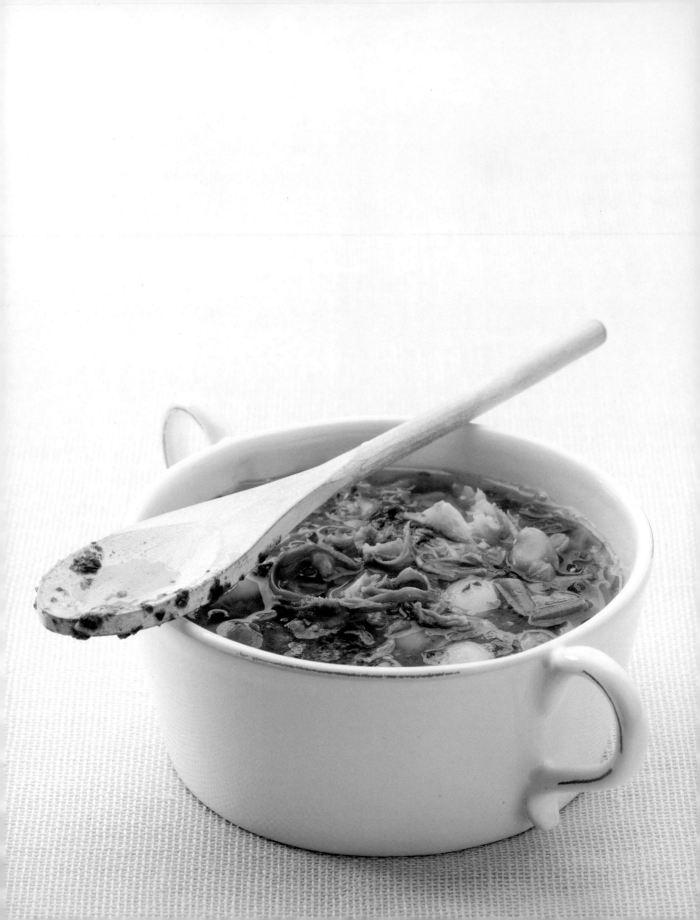

GREEN & WHITE BEAN SOUP WITH PARMA HAM

PREPARATION TIME 20 minutes, plus soaking the beans overnight and making the stock

COOKING TIME 1½ hours

200g/7oz/1 cup dried butter/lima beans

2 tbsp fruity extra-virgin olive oil, plus extra to serve

4 large garlic cloves, finely chopped

1 leek, thinly sliced and rinsed

1 onion, chopped

1.4l/48fl oz/6 cups Vegetable Stock (see page 12) or ready-made stock

1 small handful of sage and ½ celery stalk with its leaves, tied together

1 heel of Parma ham/prosciutto (see page 9; optional)

¼ head Savoy cabbage, cored and shredded

85g/3oz/½ cup chopped green beans

85g/3oz/½ cup shelled broad/fava beans, peeled if not young and tender

1 handful of baby spinach leaves

salt and freshly ground black pepper

pesto, to serve (optional)

Put the butter/lima beans in a bowl, cover with water and leave to soak overnight, then drain.

Heat the oil in a saucepan over a mediumheat. Stir in the garlic, leek and onion, reduce the heat to low and cook, covered, for 10–12 minutes, stirring occasionally, until softened but not coloured. Stir in the butter/lima beans and stock, cover and bring to the boil. Skim, then reduce the heat, stir in the sage and ham heel, if using, and simmer, covered, for 40 minutes–1 hour until tender.

Remove the ham heel and set aside until cool enough to handle. Add the cabbage, green beans and broad/fava beans to the pan and simmer, uncovered, for 10–12 minutes until all the beans are tender. Stir in the spinach and simmer for another 1 minute until the leaves wilt.

Remove the meat from the ham heel, shred it into small pieces and set aside. Season the soup with salt and pepper, but remember the ham heel will have been salty. Serve with the ham sprinkled over the top, if used. Add a dollop of pesto to each portion, if using, and serve with olive oil on the side for drizzling.

WINTER MINESTRONE

PREPARATION TIME 20 minutes, plus overnight soaking and cooking the beans

COOKING TIME 45 minutes

100g/3½oz/½ cup dried cannellini beans

140g/5oz pancetta, skinned, if necessary, and chopped

1 large onion, finely chopped

4 large garlic cloves, chopped

100g/3½oz/1½ cups finely shredded white cabbage

1 carrot, peeled, halved lengthways and sliced

1 courgette/zucchini, halved lengthways and sliced

1 floury/russet potato, peeled and chopped

1 Parmesan cheese rind, about 7.5 x 5cm/ 3 x 2in (see page 9)

100g/3½oz/½ cup Arborio rice

salt and freshly ground black pepper

extra-virgin olive oil, to serve

freshly grated Parmesan cheese, to serve (optional)

Put the beans in a bowl, cover with water and leave to soak overnight, then drain. Transfer to a saucepan, add 1.5l/52fl oz/6½ cups water, cover and bring to the boil. Reduce the heat and simmer, covered, for 50 minutes–1 hour until almost tender, then drain.

Put the pancetta in a saucepan over a medium-high heat and fry, stirring, until the fat runs. Add the onion and fry, stirring, for 5–8 minutes until softened and turning golden. Add the garlic, cabbage, carrot, courgette/zucchini and potato and stir for 1–2 minutes. Add the cheese rind and 1.5l/52fl oz/6½ cups water.

Cover and bring to the boil. Season with salt and pepper but remember the rind is salty. Reduce the heat and simmer, covered, for 10 minutes. Stir in the cooked dried beans and rice, return the soup to the boil, uncovered, then reduce the heat slightly and slowly boil for 10–15 minutes until the beans and rice are tender. Discard the cheese rind, then adjust the salt and pepper, if necessary. Serve with oil and cheese, if using.

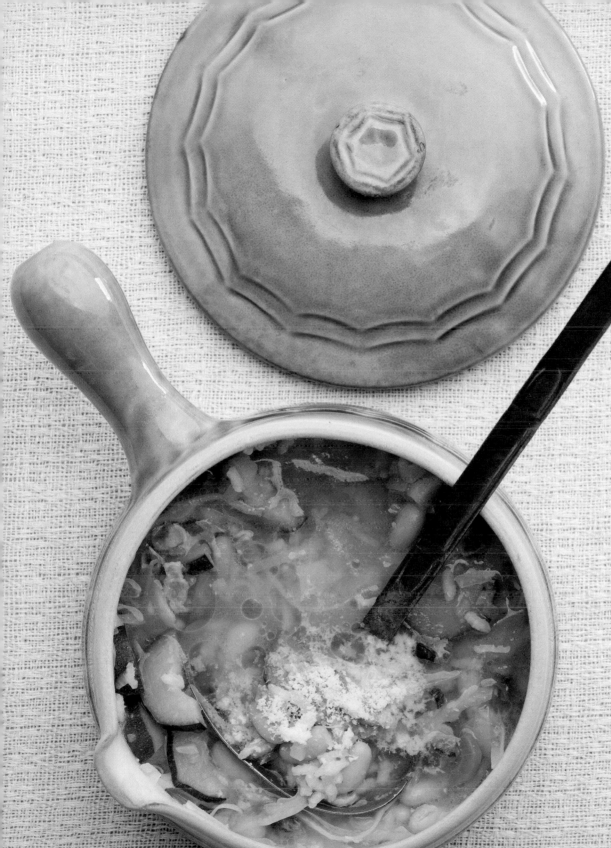

THAI MEATBALL & COCONUT SOUP

PREPARATION TIME 25 minutes, plus making the stock, chillies and garlic
COOKING TIME 20 minutes

400g/14oz minced/ground pork

2 coriander/cilantro sprigs, leaves and stalks very finely chopped, plus an extra handful of leaves, chopped

2.5cm/1in piece of fresh ginger, peeled and very finely chopped

1½ tbsp cornflour/cornstarch

1 tbsp sesame oil

1 tbsp light soy sauce or tamari soy sauce

1l/35fl oz/4½ cups Vegetable Stock (see page 12) or ready-made stock

400ml/14fl oz/1¾ cups coconut milk

1½ tbsp fish sauce, or to taste

salt and freshly ground black pepper

finely grated zest of 1 lime, to serve

Crisp-Fried Garlic (see page 19), to serve

Chillies in Vinegar (see page 19), to serve

Put the pork, finely chopped coriander/cilantro, ginger, cornflour/cornstarch, sesame oil and soy sauce in a large bowl and season with salt and pepper. Use your hands to mix together and divide the mixture into 6 equal portions, then divide each one into 6 portions to make a total of 36. Roll into meatballs and set aside.

Put the stock in a saucepan, cover and bring to the boil, then reduce the heat so the liquid boils only very lightly. Working in batches, if necessary, to avoid overcrowding the pan, add the meatballs and cook, uncovered, for 3–5 minutes until they pop to the surface and are cooked through if you cut one open. Remove the cooked meatballs from the pan and set aside. Reserve the cooking liquid.

Put the coconut milk and fish sauce in another saucepan and bring to just below the boil. Season with salt and pepper, add the meatballs and slowly stir in enough of the meatball cooking liquid to achieve the preferred consistency. Stir in the chopped coriander/cilantro leaves, adjust the salt and pepper, if necessary, and add more fish sauce, if you like. Divide the meatballs and soup into bowls and sprinkle with the lime zest. Serve with the garlic and chillies on the side.

POSOLE

PREPARATION TIME 15 minutes, plus overnight soaking
and cooking the hominy and making the stock

COOKING TIME 1¾ hours

280g/10oz/2 cups hominy (dried corn kernels)

2l/70fl oz/2 quarts Chicken Stock (see page 12) or ready-made stock

1kg/2¼lb boneless pork shoulder, in one piece, rind and fat removed

any available pork bones (optional; ask the butcher for these)

2 large onions, unpeeled, quartered and each piece studded with 1 clove

4 large garlic cloves, chopped

1 tbsp dried oregano

2 tsp ground cumin

2 green jalapeño chillies, deseeded (optional) and sliced

2 tbsp dried thyme leaves

1 tsp dried ancho chilli powder

1 tsp salt, plus extra to season

freshly ground black pepper

1 handful of coriander/cilantro leaves, chopped, to serve

Put the hominy in a bowl, cover with water and leave to soak overnight, then drain. Transfer to a saucepan and cover generously with water. Cover and bring to the boil, then reduce the heat and simmer for 4 hours. Drain and set aside.

Put the stock, pork and pork bones, if using, in a saucepan. Cover and bring to the boil. Skim, then add the onions, garlic, oregano and cumin. Reduce the heat and simmer, covered, for 30 minutes.

Add the hominy, chillies, thyme, chilli powder and salt. Cover and return to the boil, then reduce the heat and simmer for another 1–1¼ hours until the meat and hominy are very tender. Remove the pork and set aside until cool enough to handle. Discard the onions and bones, if used.

Shred the pork, then return it to the pan. Adjust the salt and pepper, if necessary, and serve sprinkled with coriander/cilantro.

PORTUGUESE CALDO VERDE

PREPARATION TIME 10 minutes

COOKING TIME 30 minutes

500g/1lb 2oz floury/russet potatoes, peeled and chopped

2 large garlic cloves, chopped

250g/9oz/3½ cups shredded curly kale or Savoy cabbage

1 tsp dried dill or thyme leaves

100g/3½oz chorizo, casing removed and meat thinly sliced

salt and freshly ground black pepper

crusty country-style bread, to serve

fruity extra-virgin olive oil, to serve

Put the potatoes, garlic and 1.25l/44fl oz/ 5½ cups water in a saucepan and season with salt and pepper. Cover and bring to the boil. Reduce the heat and simmer, covered, for 10–15 minutes until the potatoes are very tender.

Use a potato masher or large metal spoon to coarsely mash the potatoes into the water. Add the kale and dill and simmer, uncovered, for 5–10 minutes until the kale wilts. Stir in the chorizo and warm through, then adjust the salt and pepper, if necessary. Serve with bread and olive oil for adding at the table.

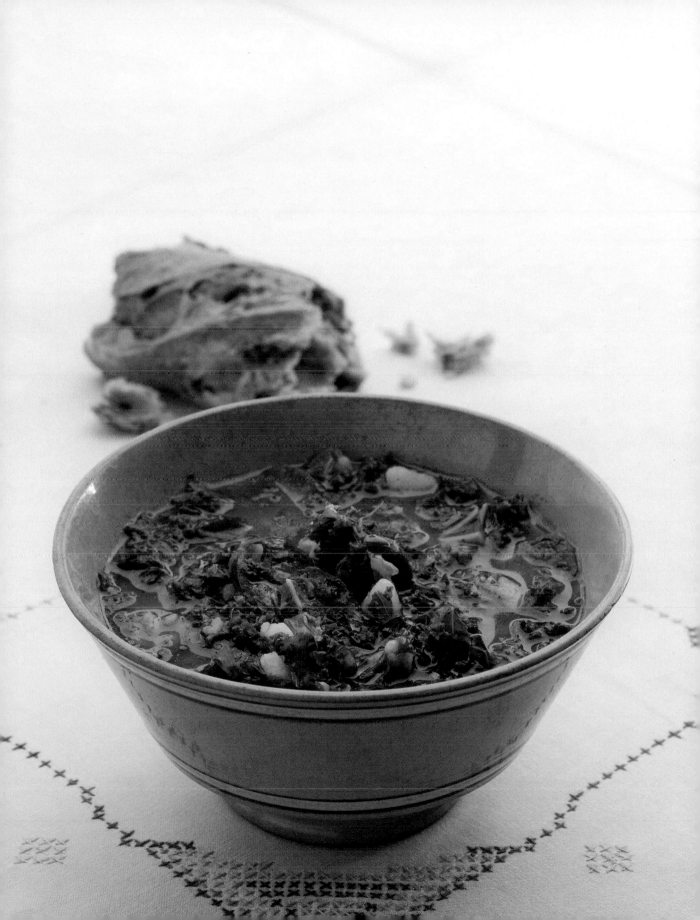

VENISON & CHESTNUT SOUP

PREPARATION TIME 25 minutes, plus making the stock and at least 4 hours marinating

COOKING TIME 1¾ hours

600g/1lb 5oz boneless venison shoulder, trimmed and cut into large chunks

240ml/8fl oz/1 cup full-flavoured dry red wine, such as Burgundy

1 shallot, sliced

1 tsp juniper berries, lightly crushed

4 large garlic cloves, chopped

1 tbsp olive oil

1 carrot, peeled and diced

1 celery stalk, chopped

½ leek, halved lengthways, thinly sliced and rinsed

1.4l/48fl oz/6 cups Beef Stock (see page 11) or ready-made stock

1 bouquet garni made with 1 piece of celery stalk, 1 bay leaf, several parsley sprigs and 2 sage sprigs tied together

½–1 tbsp redcurrant jelly (optional)

6 peeled canned or vacuum-packed chestnuts, drained and chopped

salt and freshly ground black pepper

chopped parsley leaves, to serve

Mix the venison, wine, shallot, juniper berries and half the garlic together in a non-reactive bowl. Cover and chill for at least 4 hours or up to 24.

Remove the venison from the marinade and set aside. Strain the marinade into a clean bowl and reserve.

Heat the oil in a saucepan over a medium heat. Add the carrot, celery and leek and fry, stirring occasionally, for 2 minutes. Add the remaining garlic and fry for 1–3 minutes until the leek is softened. Add the reserved marinade and cook for 8 minutes until almost evaporated. Add the stock and venison and season with salt and pepper.

Cover and bring to the boil, then skim and add the bouquet garni. Reduce the heat to very low (use a heat diffuser if you have one) and simmer, covered, for 1¼–1½ hours until the meat is very tender. Remove the venison from the soup and set aside. Discard the bouquet garni.

Stir in ½ tablespoon of the jelly, if using, then blend the soup until smooth. Return the venison to the pan, add the chestnuts and warm through. Adjust the salt and pepper, if necessary, and add more jelly, if you like. Serve sprinkled with parsley.

ROAST PHEASANT & LENTIL SOUP

PREPARATION TIME 20 minutes, plus roasting the pheasant and making the shallots

COOKING TIME 50 minutes

280g/10oz/1½ cups dried Puy or other green lentils, rinsed

2 large garlic cloves, chopped

1 leek, chopped and rinsed

1 red onion, chopped

1 tsp juniper berries and 1 bay leaf tied together in a piece of muslin/cheesecloth

400g/14oz/2½ cups finely shredded boneless, skinless roast pheasant

any leftover pheasant gravy (optional)

4 tbsp crème fraîche or sour cream

salt and freshly ground black pepper

Crisp-Fried Shallots (see page 19), to serve

chopped parsley leaves, to serve

Put the lentils, garlic, leek, onion, spice bundle and 1.75l/60fl oz/7½ cups water in a saucepan over a high heat. Cover and bring to the boil. Skim, then reduce the heat and simmer for 30–40 minutes until the lentils are very soft. Drain, reserving the cooking liquid and discarding the spice bundle.

Put a small amount of the cooking liquid in a small saucepan over a medium heat. Add the pheasant and simmer to warm through.

Meanwhile, blend the lentils with 500ml/18fl oz/2¼ cups of the cooking liquid until smooth, then season with salt and pepper. Work the soup through a sieve into a bowl, rubbing back and forth with a spoon and scraping the bottom of the sieve.

Return the soup to the pan and slowly stir in the gravy, if using, and enough of the remaining cooking liquid to achieve the preferred consistency. (Any leftover cooking liquid can be used in other recipes or frozen for up to 6 months.) Stir in the crème fraîche, then adjust the salt and pepper, if necessary. Use a slotted spoon to transfer the pheasant to the soup. Serve sprinkled with the shallots and parsley.

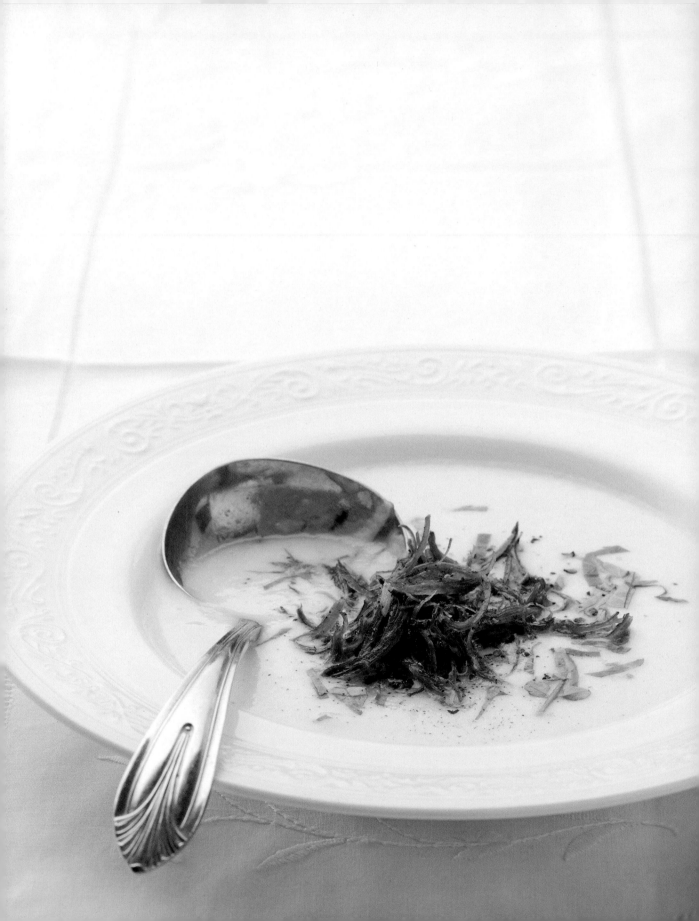

POULTRY SOUPS

The mild flavour of chicken and turkey gives cooks an almost blank canvas for creating delicious soups bursting with myriad flavours. The Thai Red Curry Chicken Soup and Mexican Chicken Noodle Soup, for example, have big, bold tastes, while the Chicken Soup with Matzo Balls and Scottish Cock-a-Leekie are more subtle, but nonetheless satisfying and sustaining. While many of the recipes in this chapter could easily become everyday stalwarts, others like the Jerusalem Artichoke Soup with Duck Confit make impressive first-course options for dinner parties.

Poultry is a favourite ingredient almost everywhere in the world, and that is reflected in the variety of recipes here. The recipe for Chicken & Sweetcorn Soup lets you recreate a restaurant favourite at home, and Chicken Gumbo Soup captures the traditional flavours of the American South.

And, of course, a homemade chicken soup can be just what the doctor ordered when you're feeling under the weather. Chicken Noodle Soup is a universal cure-all for everything from the common cold to general malaise.

CHICKEN & SWEETCORN SOUP

PREPARATION TIME 10 minutes, plus making the stock

COOKING TIME 25 minutes

2 tbsp arrowroot

1l/35fl oz/4½ cups Rich Chicken Stock (see page 11) or ready-made stock

400g/14oz boneless, skinless chicken breasts

1 can (400g/14oz) creamed sweetcorn/corn

½ tsp caster/granulated sugar

1 egg, beaten

salt and freshly ground black pepper

2 spring onions/scallions, finely chopped, to serve

Put the arrowroot and 3 tablespoons cold water in a small heatproof bowl and mix until smooth, then set aside.

Put the stock and chicken in a saucepan and season with salt and pepper. Cover and bring to the boil, then reduce the heat and simmer for 10–12 minutes until the chicken is cooked through and the juices run clear when you cut a piece. Remove the chicken from the stock and set aside until cool enough to handle.

Add the sweetcorn/corn and sugar to the pan. Stir a ladleful of the hot stock into the arrowroot mixture, then stir this mixture into the pan. Return to the boil, then boil for 2–3 minutes until the soup thickens slightly.

Meanwhile, shred the chicken, return it to the soup and reduce the heat to low. Slowly add the egg, stirring quickly with a fork until it sets in small pieces – the quicker you stir, the finer the pieces will be. Adjust the salt and pepper, if necessary, then serve sprinkled with the spring onions/scallions. If you reheat the soup, do not boil it or the eggs will scramble.

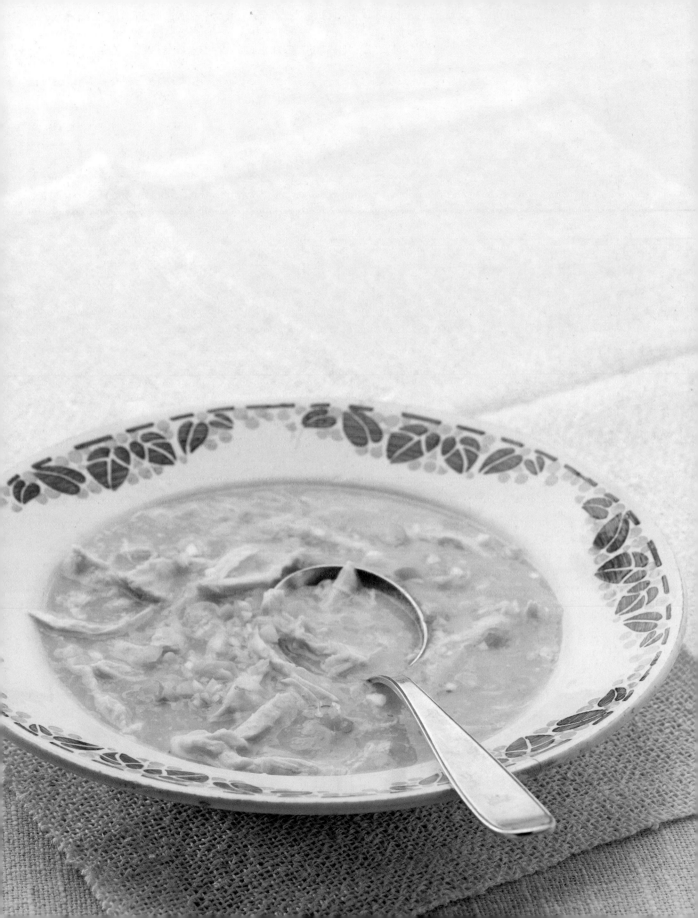

PROVENÇAL-STYLE CHICKEN SOUP

PREPARATION TIME 15 minutes, plus making the stock and croûtes
COOKING TIME 25 minutes

1 tbsp extra-virgin olive oil, plus extra to serve

1 red onion, finely chopped

4 garlic cloves, very finely chopped

700ml/24fl oz/3 cups passata (Italian sieved tomatoes)

500ml/18fl oz/2¼ cups Chicken Stock (see page 12) or ready-made stock

500g/1lb 2oz skinless chicken thighs

1 courgette/zucchini, halved lengthways and sliced

1 bouquet garni made with 1 piece of celery stalk, 1 bay leaf, several parsley and thyme sprigs and 1 rosemary sprig tied together

salt and freshly ground black pepper

chopped parsley leaves, to serve

1 recipe quantity Goats' Cheese Croûtes (see page 17), to serve

Heat the oil in a saucepan over a medium heat. Add the onion and fry for 2 minutes. Add the garlic and fry for 1–3 minutes until the onion is softened but not browned. Add the passata, stock and chicken. Cover and bring to the boil, then skim.

Add the courgette/zucchini and bouquet garni and season with salt and pepper. Reduce the heat and simmer, covered, for 10–15 minutes until the chicken is cooked through and the juices run clear when you cut a piece. Remove the chicken from the soup and set aside until cool enough to handle, then discard the bouquet garni.

Cut the chicken from the bones into bite-size pieces, return it to the soup and reheat. Adjust the salt and pepper, if necessary, then serve drizzled with oil, sprinkled with parsley and with the croûtes on the side.

CHICKEN, FENNEL & SAFFRON SOUP

PREPARATION TIME 10 minutes, plus making the stock

COOKING TIME 30 minutes

1 tbsp olive or hemp oil

280g/10oz/2 cups quartered and thinly sliced fennel, with the fronds reserved to serve

2 large garlic cloves, finely chopped

1 tsp fennel seeds

1.25l/44fl oz/5½ cups Chicken Stock (see page 12) or ready-made stock

500g/1lb 2oz skinless chicken thighs

1 bay leaf

a large pinch of saffron threads

salt and freshly ground black pepper

Heat the oil in a saucepan over a medium heat. Add the fennel and fry, stirring occasionally, for 2 minutes. Add the garlic and fry for 1–3 minutes until the fennel is softened but not coloured. Add the fennel seeds and stir for 30 seconds. Watch closely so they do not burn.

Add the stock and chicken. Cover and bring to the boil. Skim, then add the bay leaf and saffron and season with salt and pepper. Reduce the heat and simmer, covered, for 10–15 minutes until the chicken is cooked through and the juices run clear when you cut a piece. Remove the chicken from the soup and set aside until cool enough to handle.

Cut the chicken into bite-size pieces, return it to the soup and reheat. Discard the bay leaf and adjust the salt and pepper, if necessary. Serve sprinkled with the fennel fronds.

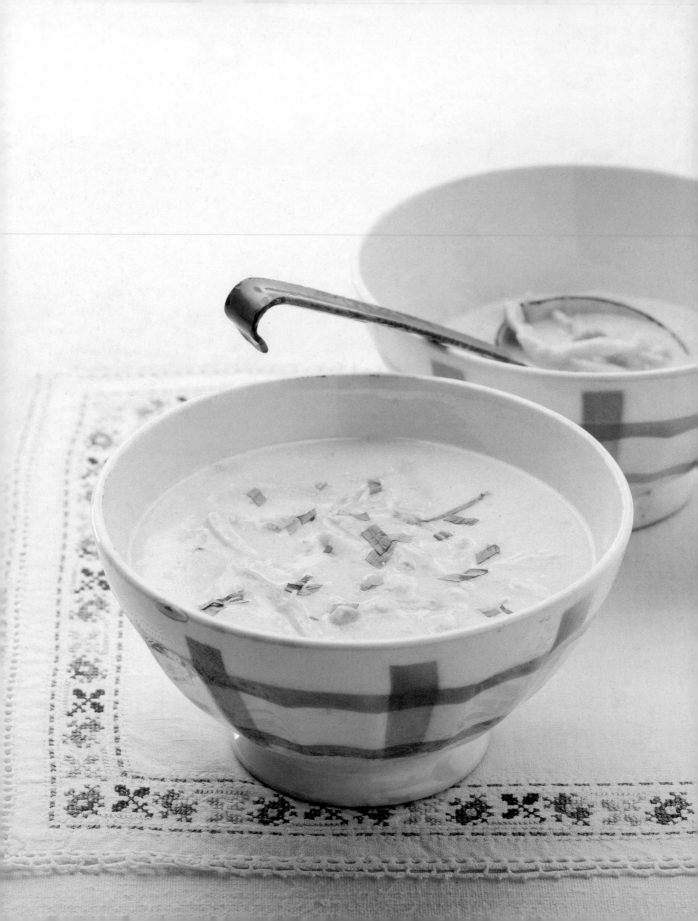

CREAM OF CHICKEN SOUP WITH TARRAGON & LEMON

PREPARATION TIME 15 minutes, plus making the stock

COOKING TIME 30 minutes

1l/35fl oz/4½ cups Rich Chicken Stock
(see page 11) or ready-made stock

500g/1lb 2oz skinless chicken thighs

4 tarragon sprigs, plus extra leaves, chopped,
to serve

1 bay leaf

1 leek, chopped and rinsed

2 tbsp butter

1 tbsp sunflower oil

2 shallots, finely chopped

4 tbsp plain white/all-purpose flour

125ml/4fl oz/½ cup double/heavy cream

finely grated zest of 1 lemon

salt and ground white pepper

Put the stock and chicken in a saucepan and season with salt and white pepper. Cover and bring to the boil, then skim. Add the tarragon, bay leaf and leek, reduce the heat and simmer, covered, for 10–15 minutes until the chicken is cooked through and the juices run clear when you cut a piece. Remove the chicken from the stock and set aside until cool enough to handle. Strain the stock and set aside.

Melt the butter with the oil in another saucepan. Add the shallots and fry, stirring occasionally, for 3–5 minutes until softened but not coloured. Sprinkle in the flour and stir for 2 minutes, then slowly add the stock, stirring continuously to prevent lumps from forming. Leave to simmer while you prepare the chicken.

Cut the chicken from the bones into thin pieces and return it to the soup. Stir in the cream and lemon zest and reheat. Adjust the salt and pepper, if necessary, then serve sprinkled with tarragon.

CHICKEN-UDON HOTPOT

PREPARATION TIME 10 minutes, plus making the stock

COOKING TIME 35 minutes

2l/70fl oz/2 quarts Chicken Stock (see page 12) or ready-made stock

750g/1lb 10oz skinless chicken thighs

2 slices of carrot for each bowl

1 shiitake mushroom cap for each bowl

400g/14oz/5 cups baby spinach leaves

3 mangetout/snow peas for each bowl

500g/1lb 2oz fresh udon noodles

salt and freshly ground black pepper

yuzu powder or grated lemon zest, to serve

togarashi seasoning, to serve (optional)

Put the stock in a saucepan over a high heat. Add the chicken and season with salt and pepper. Cover and bring to just below the boil. Skim, then reduce the heat and simmer, covered, for 15–20 minutes until the chicken is cooked through and the juices run clear when you cut a piece. Remove from the pan and set aside until cool enough to handle. Skim the excess fat from the surface of the stock, then add the carrots and shiitake mushrooms and leave to simmer.

Meanwhile, bring a separate saucepan of lightly salted water to the boil and cook the spinach for 30 seconds until it just wilts. Transfer to a colander, using a slotted spoon, and immediately rinse under cold running water, then set aside. Return the water to the boil, add the mangetout/snow peas and boil for 2–3 minutes until just tender. Drain and immediately rinse under cold running water.

Cut the chicken from the bones into bite-size pieces. Return the stock to just below the boil, add the noodles and simmer for 1–2 minutes, or according to the package instructions, to warm through.

Divide the noodles and spinach into bowls and top each portion with some of the chicken, 3 mangetout/snow peas, 2 carrot slices and 1 shiitake mushroom. Add the stock and serve sprinkled with yuzu and togarashi, if you like.

MALAY-STYLE CHICKEN SOUP

PREPARATION TIME 25 minutes, plus making the stock

COOKING TIME 45 minutes

1.4l/48fl oz/6 cups Chicken Stock (see page 12) or ready-made stock

1cm/½in piece of galangal, peeled and sliced

1cm/½in piece of fresh ginger, peeled and sliced

2 garlic cloves, crushed

2 shallots, sliced

1 bird's-eye chilli, deseeded (optional) and sliced

1 lemongrass stick, coarsely chopped, with outer leaves removed

1 floury/russet potato, peeled and chopped

500g/1lb 2oz skinless chicken thighs

140g/5oz/1 cup diced pumpkin

100g/3½oz/¾ cup chopped green beans

200ml/7fl oz/scant 1 cup coconut milk

2 tbsp lime juice, or to taste

1 tbsp fish sauce, or to taste

salt and freshly ground black pepper

chopped coriander/cilantro leaves, to serve

finely shredded spring onions/scallions, to serve

Put the stock, galangal, ginger, garlic, shallots, chilli, lemongrass and potato in a saucepan. Cover and bring to the boil, skimming as necessary. Boil, partially covered, for 15 minutes until the potato is very tender. Strain into a large bowl, pressing down on the potato to push as much as possible through the sieve, then return the stock to the pan. Discard the flavourings.

Add the chicken, pumpkin and green beans and season with pepper. Cover and bring to the boil. Reduce the heat and simmer for 10–15 minutes until the chicken is cooked through and the juices run clear when you cut a piece. Remove the chicken from the soup and set aside until cool enough to handle.

Cut the chicken from the bones and slice, then return it to the soup. Add the coconut milk, lime juice and fish sauce and simmer over a very low heat, stirring, for 2–3 minutes. Adjust the salt and pepper and add more lime juice or fish sauce, if necessary. Serve sprinkled with coriander/cilantro and spring onions/scallions.

THAI RED CURRY CHICKEN SOUP

PREPARATION TIME 15 minutes, plus making the chillies
COOKING TIME 30 minutes

2 tbsp sunflower oil

2 large shallots, sliced

1 tbsp red curry paste

500g/1lb 2oz skinless chicken thighs

400ml/14fl oz/1¾ cups coconut milk

2.5cm/1in piece of fresh ginger, peeled and sliced

4 kaffir lime leaves, torn

lime juice, to taste (optional)

palm sugar or light brown sugar, to taste (optional)

chopped coriander/cilantro leaves, to serve

Chillies in Vinegar (see page 19), to serve

lime wedges, to serve (optional)

Measure 1l/35fl oz/4½ cups water into a large measuring jug/cup and set aside.

Heat the oil in a large wok with a lid or a saucepan over a high heat. Add the shallots and curry paste, reduce the heat to medium and stir-fry for 2 minutes. Very slowly stir in 200ml/7fl oz/ scant 1 cup of the water and stir for 1–2 minutes until the fat forms bubbles on the surface. Add the chicken and fry, turning occasionally, for 5 minutes, gradually stirring in a little more of the measured water if the curry paste looks like it will burn. Slowly add the coconut milk, ginger, lime leaves and remaining water, then cover and bring to the boil.

Reduce the heat and simmer for 10–15 minutes until the chicken is cooked through and the juices run clear when you cut a piece. Remove the chicken from the soup and set aside until cool enough to handle.

Cut the chicken from the bones into bite-size pieces and return it to the soup. Stir in the lime juice and palm sugar to temper the heat of the curry paste, if you like, and reheat the soup. Serve sprinkled with coriander/cilantro, topped with chillies and with lime wedges for squeezing over, if you like.

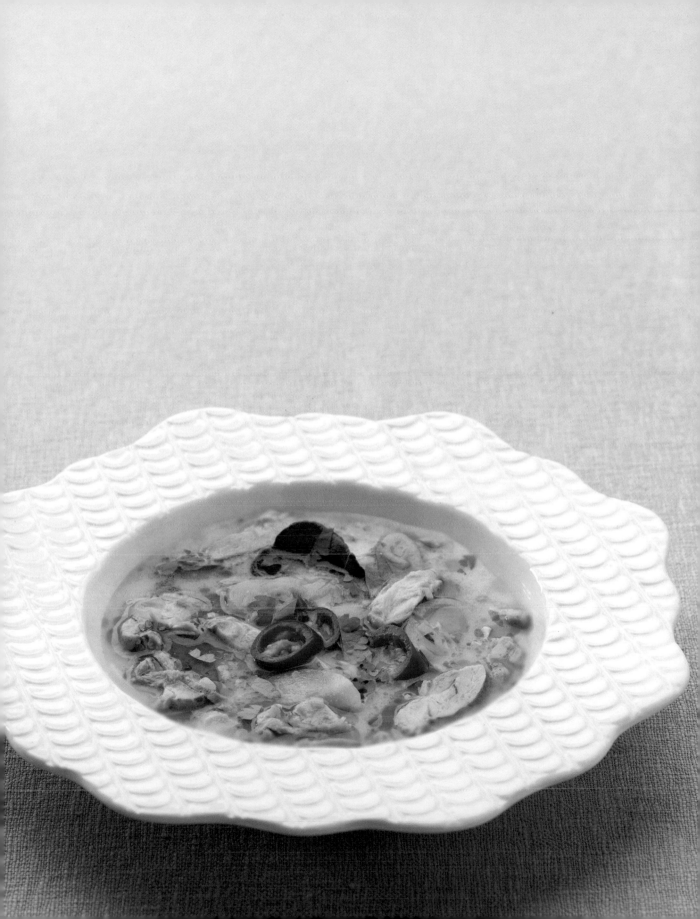

'VELVET' CHICKEN & EDAMAME SOUP

PREPARATION TIME 25 minutes, plus making the stock

COOKING TIME 20 minutes

400g/14oz boneless chicken thighs

1.4l/48fl oz/6 cups Rich Chicken Stock (see page 11) or ready-made stock

4cm/1½in piece of fresh ginger, peeled and grated

1 thin slice of galangal, peeled and smashed in one piece

100g/3½oz/¾ cup frozen shelled edamame beans (green soy beans)

½ tsp salt

100g/3½oz canned water chestnuts, drained, rinsed and finely chopped

3 spring onions/scallions, thinly sliced on the diagonal

2 tsp light soy sauce or tamari soy sauce, or to taste

Up to 2 hours in advance, prepare the chicken. Put the chicken, skin side down, on a chopping board and use the flat side of a cleaver or large chef's knife to pound it several times to flatten. Next, use the flat edge along the top of the cleaver or knife to pound the meat until it looks like it has been minced/ground, then use the sharp edge of the knife to scrape the meat away from the skin. Discard the skin. Finely chop the meat, occasionally adding 1 teaspoon cold water until it becomes almost white and fluffy. (You can add up to 3 tablespoons water.) Cover and chill until required. Alternatively, skin and very thinly slice the thighs.

When ready to cook, bring a small saucepan of water to the boil for the edamame. Put the stock in a separate saucepan, cover and bring to just below the boil. Add the ginger and galangal to the stock, reduce the heat to low, and simmer while you cook the edamame.

Add the edamame and salt to the boiling water and boil for 5 minutes until tender. Drain and immediately rinse under cold running water to stop the cooking.

Add the chicken, edamame, water chestnuts and spring onions/scallions to the stock and simmer for 2–3 minutes until the chicken is cooked through. Discard the galangal. Stir in the soy sauce, adding extra to taste, if you like, then serve.

MEXICAN CHICKEN NOODLE SOUP

PREPARATION TIME 35 minutes, plus making the stock and cooking the chicken

COOKING TIME 25 minutes

1 dried chipotle chilli pepper

2 tbsp garlic-flavoured olive oil

1 red onion, finely chopped

1 red pepper, deseeded and diced

100g/3½oz very thin egg noodles, such as vermicelli, broken into bite-size pieces

1 tsp ground cumin

1 tsp dried thyme leaves

1.25l/44fl oz/5½ cups Chicken Stock (see page 12) or ready-made stock

200ml/7fl oz/scant 1 cup passata (Italian sieved tomatoes)

a pinch of light brown sugar

400g/14oz/3 cups shredded boneless, skinless cooked chicken

salt and freshly ground black pepper

chopped coriander/cilantro leaves, to serve

hot pepper sauce, to serve

tortilla chips, to serve (optional)

Put the chipotle pepper in a bowl, cover with warm water and leave to soak for 20 minutes until tender, then drain, deseed and chop.

Heat half the oil in a saucepan. Add the onion and red pepper and fry, stirring occasionally, for 3–5 minutes until the onion is softened but not coloured. Add the remaining oil to the pan and heat. Add the noodles and fry for 2–3 minutes until they just start to brown. Add the chipotle, cumin and thyme and stir for 30 seconds until aromatic. Watch closely so the noodles do not overbrown and the spices do not burn.

Stir in the stock, passata and sugar and season with salt and pepper. Cover and bring to the boil, then boil, uncovered, for 3–5 minutes until the noodles and red pepper are tender. Stir in the chicken and warm through, and adjust the salt and pepper, if necessary. Serve sprinkled with coriander/cilantro and with hot pepper sauce and tortilla chips, if you like, on the side. If reheating this soup, add a little extra stock, if necessary, to thin it.

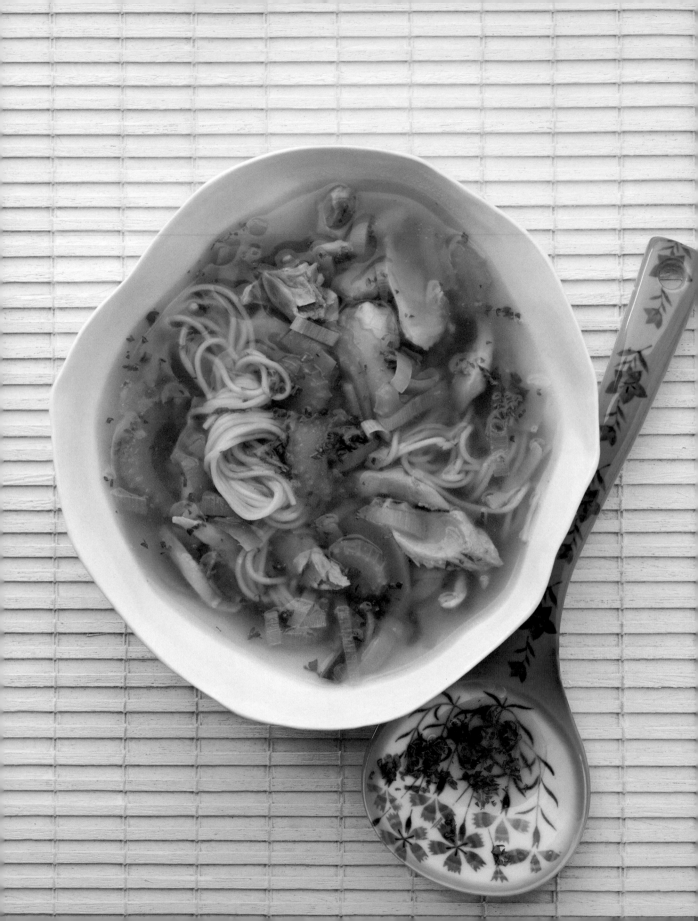

CHICKEN NOODLE SOUP

PREPARATION TIME 15 minutes, plus making the stock and cooking the chicken

COOKING TIME 25 minutes

1.25l/44fl oz/5½ cups Rich Chicken Stock
(see page 11)

500g/1lb 2oz skinless chicken drumsticks and/
or thighs, or 400g/14oz/3 cups chicken from
making the stock, cut into bite-size pieces

2 carrots, peeled and sliced

2 celery stalks, sliced

1 leek, thinly sliced and rinsed

225g/8oz thin egg noodles or spaghetti

4 tbsp finely chopped parsley leaves

salt and freshly ground black pepper

If using raw chicken, put the stock in a saucepan, add the raw chicken and season with salt and pepper. Cover and bring to just below the boil. Skim, then reduce the heat and simmer, covered, for 10–15 minutes for thighs and 15–20 minutes for drumsticks until the chicken is cooked through and the juices run clear when you cut a piece. Remove the chicken from the stock and set aside until cool enough to handle. Meanwhile, bring a separate large pan of salted water to the boil.

Add the carrots, celery and leek to the stock and return to the boil. Reduce the heat and simmer for 10–12 minutes until tender.

Meanwhile, add the noodles to the boiling water and cook for 10 minutes, or according to the package instructions, until tender. Drain, rinse under cold running water and set aside.

Cut the chicken meat from the bones and into bite-size pieces. Add the freshly cooked or leftover chicken to the soup, stir in the noodles and simmer gently to reheat. Adjust the salt and pepper, if necessary, stir in the parsley and serve.

CHICKEN, PEPPER & RICE SOUP

PREPARATION TIME 15 minutes, plus making the stock and rice
COOKING TIME 30 minutes

1 tbsp garlic-flavoured olive oil

1 onion, finely chopped

1.25l/44fl oz/5½ cups Chicken Stock (see page 12) or ready-made stock

500g/1lb 2oz skinless chicken thighs

1 green pepper, deseeded and finely chopped

1 red pepper, deseeded and finely chopped

a pinch of dried chilli/hot pepper flakes, or to taste (optional)

85g/3oz/½ cup frozen sweetcorn/corn kernels

200g/7oz/1 cup long-grain rice, cooked

salt and freshly ground black pepper

chopped coriander/cilantro or parsley leaves, to serve

Heat the oil in a saucepan over a medium heat. Add the onion and fry, stirring occasionally, for 3–5 minutes until softened but not coloured. Add the stock and chicken and season with salt and pepper. Cover and bring to the boil. Skim, then reduce the heat and simmer, covered, for 5 minutes.

Add the peppers and chilli/hot pepper flakes, if using, and simmer, covered, for another 5–10 minutes until the peppers are tender and the chicken is cooked through and the juices run clear when you cut a piece. Remove the chicken from the soup and set aside until cool enough to handle.

Add the sweetcorn/corn kernels to the pan, bring to a slow boil and boil for 3–5 minutes until tender. Cut the chicken from the bones into bite-size pieces, return it to the soup with the rice and heat through. Adjust the salt and pepper, if necessary, then serve sprinkled with coriander/cilantro.

PERUVIAN 'BREAKFAST' SOUP – FOR ANY TIME OF THE DAY

PREPARATION TIME 15 minutes, plus making the stock and hard-boiling the eggs
COOKING TIME 45 minutes

1 egg for each bowl

2l/70fl oz/2 quarts Rich Chicken Stock (see page 11) or ready-made stock

6 garlic cloves, crushed

3 celery stalks, coarsely chopped

4cm/1½in piece of fresh ginger, peeled and coarsely chopped

1kg/2¼lb skinless chicken pieces, such as breasts and drumsticks

400g/14oz waxy potatoes, peeled and chopped

salt and freshly ground black pepper

chopped coriander/cilantro leaves, to serve

2 roasted red peppers in olive oil, drained and sliced, to serve

chopped spring onions/scallions, to serve

Put the eggs in a saucepan, add enough water to cover by 2.5cm/1in and bring to the boil, then reduce the heat and simmer for 9 minutes. Pour off the hot water, then run cold water over the eggs for 1–2 minutes to stop the cooking. Set aside until cool enough to handle, then peel and set aside.

Meanwhile, put the stock, garlic, celery and ginger in a saucepan and season with salt and pepper. Cover and bring to the boil, then boil, uncovered, for 10 minutes until slightly reduced. Discard the flavourings.

Add the chicken and potatoes to the pan, cover and bring to the boil. Skim, then reduce the heat and simmer for 15–20 minutes until the potatoes are tender and the chicken is cooked through and the juices run clear when you cut a piece. Remove the chicken from the pan and set aside until cool enough to handle.

Cut the chicken from the bones into bite-size pieces and return to the stock to warm through. Adjust the salt and pepper, if necessary. Cut the hard-boiled eggs in half lengthways and arrange on a plate. Serve the soup sprinkled with coriander/cilantro and with the peppers, eggs and spring onions/scallions on the side.

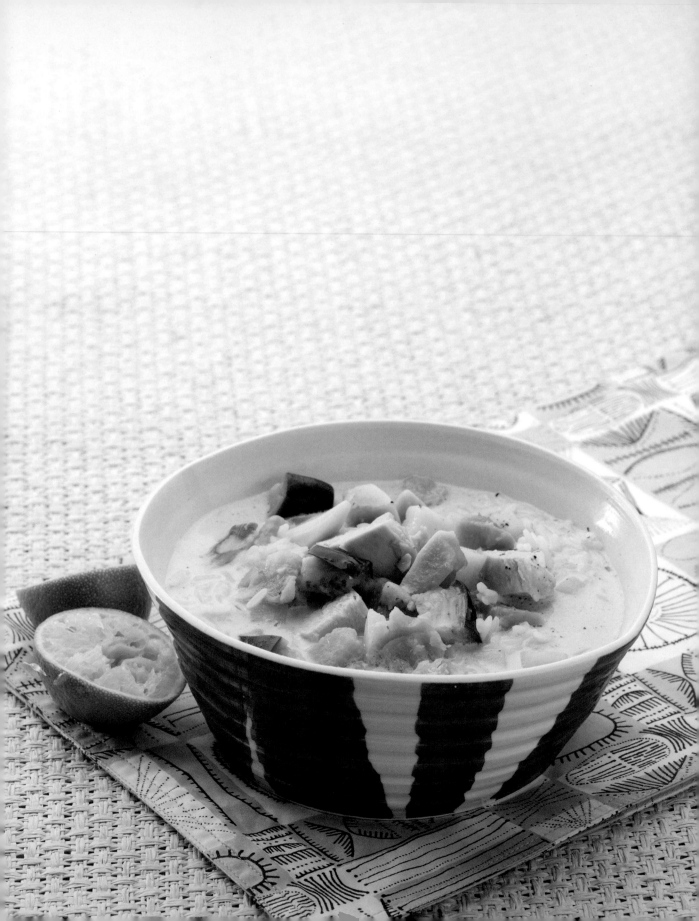

HOT, HOT, HOT CARIBBEAN CHICKEN SOUP

PREPARATION TIME 25 minutes, plus making the stock and rice and overnight chilling (optional)
COOKING TIME 45 minutes

3 tbsp sunflower oil

1 onion, chopped

2 garlic cloves, crushed

½ tsp black mustard seeds

½ tsp ground coriander

1 Scotch bonnet chilli, left whole or chopped, as desired

1.5l/52fl oz/6½ cups Chicken Stock (see page 12) or ready-made stock

750g/1lb 10oz boneless, skinless pieces of chicken, such as breasts, drumsticks and thighs

250g/9oz/2 cups peeled and deseeded butternut squash cut into bite-size pieces

3 waxy new potatoes, diced

2 bay leaves

½ aubergine/eggplant, cut into bite-size pieces

400ml/14fl oz/1¾ cups coconut milk

½ tbsp tamarind paste

1 mango, peeled, pitted and diced

1 papaya, peeled, deseeded and chopped

juice of 1 lime, plus lime wedges, to serve

salt

400g/14oz/2 cups cooked long-grain rice, hot, to serve

This soup is best made a day in advance and chilled so the excess fat can be removed. Heat the oil in a large saucepan over a medium heat. Add the onion and fry, stirring occasionally, for 7 minutes. Add the garlic and fry for 1–3 minutes until the onion is golden brown. Stir in the mustard seeds, coriander and chilli and stir for 30 seconds. Watch closely so the spices do not burn.

Add the stock, chicken, squash, potatoes, bay leaves and aubergine/eggplant and season with salt. Cover and bring to the boil. Skim, then stir in the coconut milk and tamarind paste. Reduce the heat and simmer, covered, for 15–20 minutes until the chicken is cooked through and the juices run clear when you cut a piece. Remove the chicken from the pan and set aside until cool enough to handle.

Skim the fat from the surface of the soup. (At this point, the soup can be left to cool completely, then covered and chilled overnight so the excess fat can be removed before serving.)

Add the mango, papaya and lime juice to the pan and simmer for 5 minutes. Cut the chicken into bite-size pieces and return it to the soup. Adjust the salt, if necessary, then discard the bay leaves. Serve immediately over rice and with lime wedges for squeezing over.

CHICKEN MULLIGATAWNY SOUP

PREPARATION TIME 20 minutes, plus making the stock and cooking the chicken and rice (optional)
COOKING TIME 35 minutes

1 tbsp sunflower or groundnut/peanut oil

1 apple, peeled, cored and chopped

1 carrot, peeled and chopped

1 celery stalk, thinly sliced

1 onion, finely chopped

1 green or red pepper, deseeded and chopped

1 tbsp plain white/all-purpose or wholemeal/wholewheat flour

1 tsp curry powder

½ tsp mustard powder

1.25l/44fl oz/5½ cups Rich Chicken Stock (see page 11) or ready-made stock

400g/14oz/3 cups boneless, skinless cooked chicken cut into bite-size pieces

salt and freshly ground black pepper

cooked white or brown basmati rice, hot, to serve (optional)

chopped coriander/cilantro or parsley leaves, to serve

Heat the oil in a saucepan over a medium heat. Add the apple, carrot, celery, onion and pepper and fry, stirring occasionally, for 3–5 minutes until the vegetables are softened. Sprinkle in the flour, curry powder and mustard and stir for 2 minutes. Slowly add the stock, stirring continuously to prevent lumps from forming.

Season with salt and pepper, cover and bring to the boil. Reduce the heat and simmer for 20 minutes until the apple breaks down, the vegetables are tender and the soup has thickened slightly. Add the chicken and heat through, then adjust the salt and pepper, if necessary.

Put a portion of hot rice, if using, in each bowl. Ladle the soup over it, sprinkle with coriander/cilantro and serve.

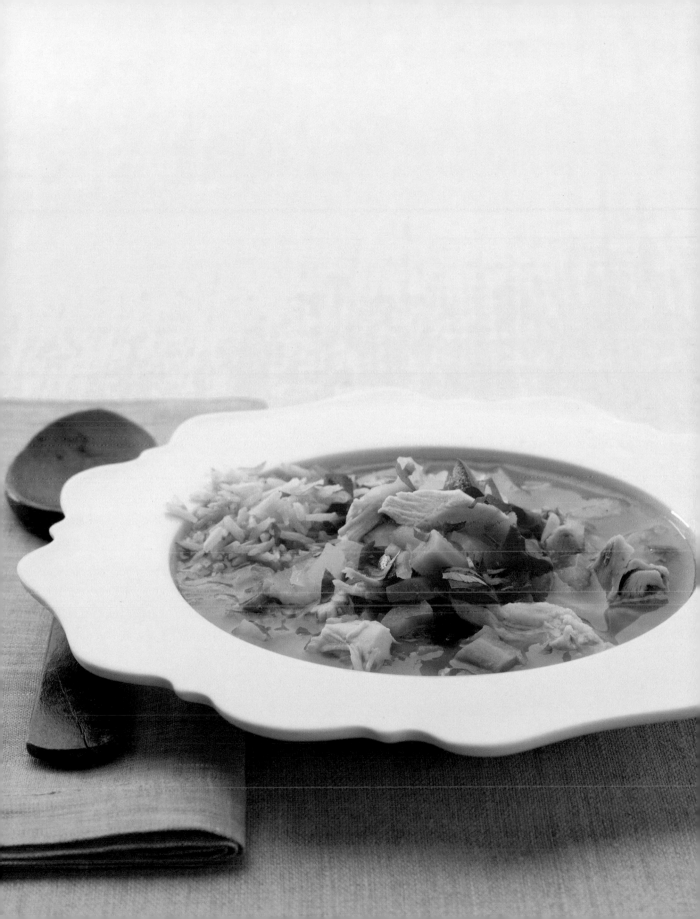

CHICKEN SOUP WITH MATZO BALLS

PREPARATION TIME 25 minutes, plus 2 hours chilling and making the stock
COOKING TIME 1¼ hours

1.25l/44fl oz/5½ cups Rich Chicken Stock
(see page 11)
1 large carrot, peeled and sliced
1 leek, halved lengthways, sliced and rinsed
115g/4oz/1½ cups shredded Savoy cabbage
salt and freshly ground black pepper
chopped parsley leaves, to serve

MATZO BALLS
2 large/extra-large eggs
2 tbsp butter, at room temperature
100g/3½oz/1 cup ground almonds
100g/3½oz/1 cup medium ground matzo meal
4–5 tbsp Rich Chicken Stock (see page 11)
or ready-made stock
olive oil, if required (optional)

To make the matzo balls, put the eggs in a large bowl and beat with an electric mixer or a wooden spoon for 2–3 minutes until very thick and pale and they hold a 'ribbon' on the surface when the mixer is lifted. Beat in the butter, almonds and matzo meal and season with salt and pepper. Gradually add the stock until the mixture is quite thick and sticky. Cover with cling film/plastic wrap and chill for 2 hours.

Bring a large saucepan of water to the boil. Using a wet spoon, divide the matzo ball mixture into 24 equal portions. Use wet hands to roll each portion into a ball. Drop the balls into the water and, just before the water returns to the boil, reduce the heat to low. Simmer for 45 minutes until the matzo balls are cooked through when you cut one open. Gently drain and set aside. If making in advance, rub the balls lightly with oil to prevent them from sticking together.

Put the stock in a saucepan. Cover and bring to just below the boil. Add the carrot and leek and season with salt and pepper. Simmer, covered, for 10 minutes, then gently stir in the matzo balls and cabbage and simmer for another 5 minutes until they are heated through and the carrots are very tender. Adjust the salt and pepper, if necessary, and serve sprinkled with parsley.

COLOMBIAN CHICKEN & CORN SOUP

PREPARATION TIME 15 minutes, plus making the stock

COOKING TIME 40 minutes

1½ tbsp sunflower oil

1 large onion, finely chopped

2 tsp dried oregano

500g/1lb 2oz skinless chicken thighs

1.25l/44fl oz/5½ cups Chicken Stock
(see page 12) or ready-made stock

1 floury/russet potato, peeled and grated

1 waxy potato, peeled and diced

3 sweetcorn/corn cobs, husked and each cut
into 2 or 3 pieces

salt and freshly ground black pepper

TO SERVE

2 avocados

1 tbsp lemon juice

chopped coriander/cilantro leaves

3 tbsp capers, rinsed

double/heavy cream

Heat the oil in a saucepan over a medium heat. Add the onion and fry, stirring, for 3–5 minutes until softened. Stir in the oregano, chicken, stock and grated potato and season with salt and pepper. Cover and bring to the boil, then reduce the heat and simmer for 10–15 minutes until the chicken is cooked through. Remove the chicken from the pan and set aside until cool enough to handle.

Add the diced potato and sweetcorn/corn to the pan, cover and return to the boil. Reduce the heat and simmer for 10–12 minutes until the vegetables are tender.

Meanwhile, peel, pit and chop the avocados and toss with the lemon juice, then set aside. Remove the chicken from the bones and cut it into bite-size pieces, return it to the soup and heat through. Adjust the salt and pepper, if necessary. Divide the sweetcorn/corn pieces into bowls and ladle the soup over them. Serve sprinkled with coriander/cilantro and with the avocado, capers and cream on the side.

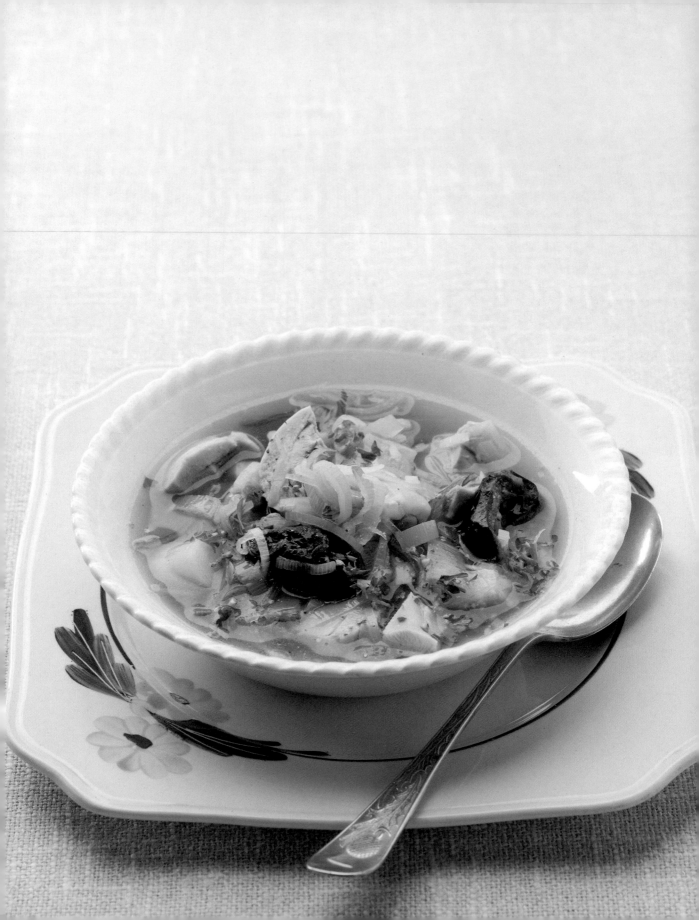

SCOTTISH COCK-A-LEEKIE

PREPARATION TIME 10 minutes, plus making
the stock

COOKING TIME 40 minutes

2 leeks, trimmed, white and green parts separated
2 tbsp butter
1.4l/48fl oz/6 cups Chicken Stock (see page 12)
500g/1lb 2oz skinless chicken thighs
1 bouquet garni made with 1 bay leaf, several
    parsley sprigs and 1 thyme sprig tied together
6 prunes, pitted and halved
chopped parsley leaves, to serve

Slice the white parts of the leeks thickly, then rinse
and set aside. Quarter the green parts lengthways
and finely shred, then rinse and set aside.

Melt the butter in a saucepan over a medium heat.
Add the white parts of the leeks and fry, stirring
occasionally, for 5–8 minutes until just starting to
turn golden. Add the stock and chicken, cover
and bring to just below the boil. Skim, then add
the bouquet garni and reduce the heat to low.
Simmer, covered, for 10–15 minutes until the
chicken is cooked through. Remove the chicken
and set aside until cool enough to handle.

Add the prunes and green parts of the leeks to the
soup and simmer, uncovered, for 5–10 minutes
until the prunes are tender. Discard the bouquet
garni. Cut the chicken from the bones into bite-size
pieces, return it to the soup and reheat. Adjust the
seasoning, then serve sprinkled with parsley.

TURKEY & RICE SOUP

PREPARATION TIME 10 minutes, plus making
the stock and cooking the turkey

COOKING TIME 35 minutes

1.4l/48fl oz/6 cups Turkey Stock (see page 12)
    or ready-made stock
2 celery stalks, halved
a pinch of dried chilli/hot pepper flakes, or
    to taste
85g/3oz/⅓ cup long-grain white rice
100g/3½oz/⅔ cup frozen sweetcorn/
    corn kernels
140g/5oz/2 cups shredded Savoy cabbage
200g/7oz/1½ cups boneless, skinless cooked
    turkey cut into bite-size pieces
1 roasted red pepper in olive oil, drained and
    finely chopped
2 tbsp chopped parsley leaves
salt and freshly ground black pepper

Put the stock, celery and chilli/hot pepper flakes
in a saucepan and season with salt and pepper.
Cover, bring to the boil and boil for 10 minutes,
then discard the celery.

Cover and return the stock to the boil. Add the
rice and boil, uncovered, for 10 minutes. Stir in
the sweetcorn/corn and cabbage and continue
boiling for 5 minutes until the rice is tender. Stir
in the turkey, red pepper and parsley and warm
through. Adjust the salt and pepper, if necessary,
and serve.

CHICKEN GUMBO SOUP

PREPARATION TIME 20 minutes, plus making the stock and rice

COOKING TIME 1½ hours

55g/2oz/¼ cup butter

2 tbsp sunflower oil

4 tbsp plain white/all-purpose flour

4 garlic cloves, finely chopped

1 large onion, finely chopped

1 green pepper, deseeded and chopped

1 red pepper, deseeded and chopped

1 celery stalk, thinly sliced

1.5l/52fl oz/6½ cups Chicken Stock (see page 12) or ready-made stock

200g/7oz/2 cups chopped okra

2 bay leaves

2 tbsp chopped parsley

1 tsp dried thyme leaves

2 cans (800g/1¾lb) chopped tomatoes

½ tsp sugar

cayenne pepper, to taste

1kg/2¼lb skinless chicken thighs

salt and freshly ground black pepper

400g/14oz/2 cups cooked long-grain rice, hot, to serve

hot pepper sauce, to serve

First, make a roux: melt the butter with the oil in a saucepan over a low heat (use a heat diffuser if you have one). Sprinkle in the flour and cook, stirring, for 15–20 minutes until it turns a deep golden brown. Watch closely because when the roux starts to brown it will colour very quickly.

Add the garlic, onion, peppers and celery and stir for 5–8 minutes until the onion is softened. Add half the stock, stirring continuously to prevent lumps from forming. Add the remaining stock, okra, bay leaves, parsley, thyme, tomatoes, sugar and cayenne pepper and season with salt and pepper. Cover and bring to the boil, then reduce the heat and simmer for 45 minutes. The okra will make the soup glutinous.

Add the chicken, cover and bring to the boil, then skim. Reduce the heat and simmer for 10–15 minutes until the chicken is cooked through and the juices run clear when you cut a piece. Remove the chicken and set aside until cool enough to handle, then cut the meat from the bones into bite-size pieces and return it to the soup. Discard the bay leaves. Reheat, adjust the salt and pepper, if necessary, and serve over the rice with the hot pepper sauce.

DUCK IN GINGER BROTH

PREPARATION TIME 25 minutes

COOKING TIME 1¼ hours

7.5cm/3in piece of fresh ginger, peeled and sliced

4 coriander/cilantro sprigs, roots and stalks coarsely chopped, with the leaves reserved to serve

2 carrots, peeled and thickly sliced, plus an extra ½ carrot, peeled and cut into matchsticks

2 large garlic cloves, chopped

2 star anise

1 large onion, unpeeled and halved

1 large leek, half thickly sliced and rinsed, and the rest cut into matchsticks and rinsed

400g/14oz boneless, skinless duck breasts

4 shiitake mushroom caps, thinly sliced

2 Chinese cabbage leaves, rolled and thinly sliced

2 spring onions/scallions, sliced on the diagonal

light soy sauce or tamari soy sauce, to taste

Put the ginger, coriander/cilantro, sliced carrots, garlic, star anise, onion, sliced leek and 1.5l/52fl oz/6½ cups water in a large saucepan. Cover and bring to the boil, then boil, uncovered, for 10 minutes to reduce slightly.

Reduce the heat to low. Add the duck and slowly return the liquid to just below the boil, skimming as necessary. Just before the liquid boils, reduce the heat to very low (use a heat diffuser if you have one) and simmer, covered, for 40–45 minutes until the duck is very tender. Remove the duck from the soup and set aside until cool enough to handle.

Strain the stock into a bowl and discard the flavourings. Return the stock to the washed pan, cover and return to the boil. Thinly slice the duck and set aside.

Reduce the heat to a simmer, then add the carrot and leek matchsticks, mushrooms, cabbage and spring onions/scallions and simmer for 5–8 minutes until they are all tender. Return the duck to the pan and reheat. Season with soy sauce and serve sprinkled with coriander/cilantro leaves.

JERUSALEM ARTICHOKE SOUP
WITH DUCK CONFIT

PREPARATION TIME 20 minutes

COOKING TIME 50 minutes

800g/1¾lb Jerusalem artichokes, unpeeled but well scrubbed

3 lemon slices

2 tbsp butter

1 large onion, finely chopped

500ml/18fl oz/2¼ cups whole milk

400g/14oz duck confit, skin and bones removed and meat finely shredded, with a little of the surrounding fat reserved

150ml/5fl oz/⅔ cup single/light cream

1½ tbsp lemon juice

salt and ground white pepper

finely shredded watercress leaves, to serve

Put the artichokes, lemon slices and 750ml/26fl oz/3¼ cups water in a saucepan, adding extra water, if needed, to cover the artichokes. Cover and bring to the boil, then reduce the heat and simmer for 20–25 minutes until the artichokes are tender but still holding their shape. Drain, reserving 600ml/20fl oz/2½ cups of the cooking liquid, and set the artichokes aside until cool enough to handle.

Use your fingers to peel the artichokes, then mash them with a fork and set aside.

Melt the butter in the washed and dried pan over a medium heat. Add the onion and fry, stirring occasionally, for 3–5 minutes until softened. Stir in the artichokes, milk and reserved cooking liquid and season with salt and white pepper. Cover and bring to just below the boil, then reduce the heat and simmer for 5 minutes. Meanwhile, heat the duck with a little of its fat in a small frying pan over a medium heat.

Blend the soup until smooth and reheat, if necessary. Stir in the cream and 1 tablespoon of the lemon juice, then adjust the salt and pepper and add extra lemon juice, if necessary. Serve sprinkled with watercress and topped with the duck confit.

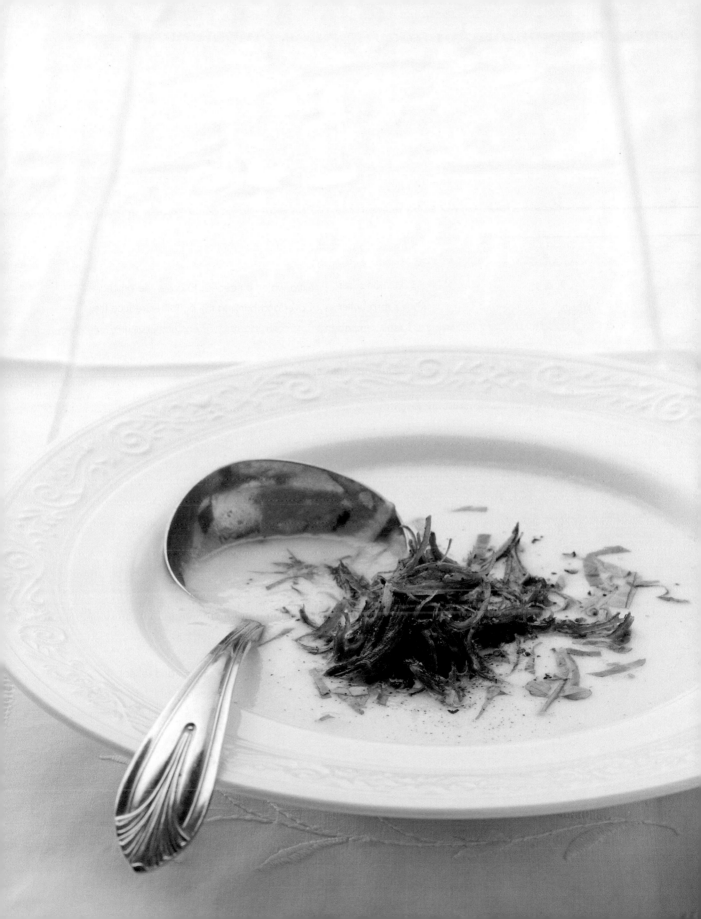

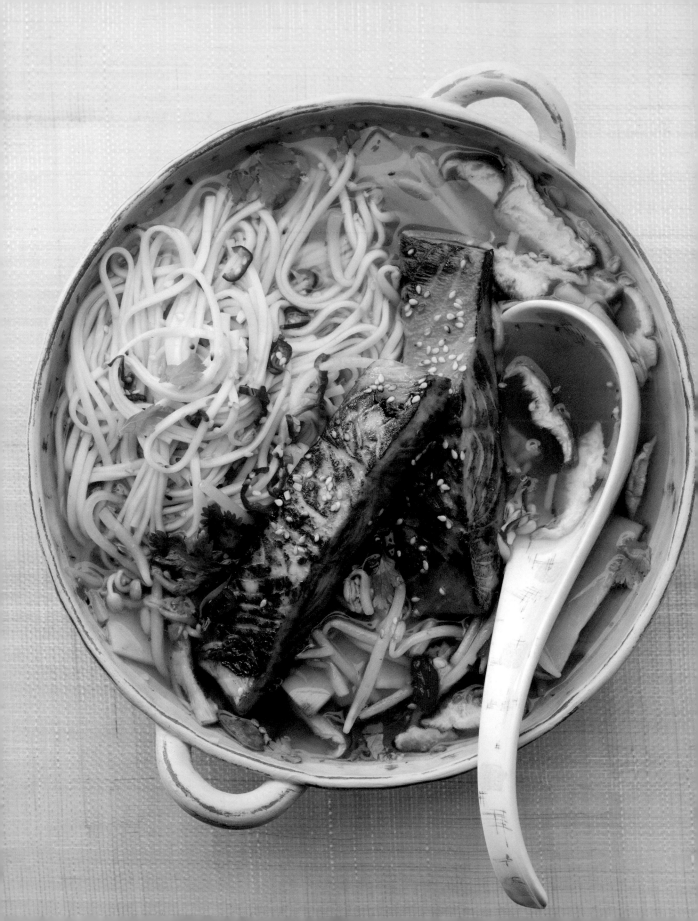

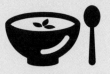

FISH &
SHELLFISH SOUPS

Seafood soups range from simple to extravagant, but they all have an essential common feature: for optimum results they must contain the freshest, best-quality fish and shellfish.

This chapter features global recipes with varied flavours and textures. Bouillabaisse and Soupe de Poissons capture the flavours of the Mediterranean, while New England Clam Chowder is an all-American favourite. From Asia, Teriyaki Salmon Ramen is a meal in a bowl, and Elegant Japanese Scallop Soup and Mackerel in Chilli-Lime Broth are stylish recipes for special occasions. You'll also find soups from the Caribbean, the Aegean, Spain, Scotland and the North Sea harbours of Scandinavia.

Top-quality seafood is generally an expensive ingredient, but for a purse-friendly treat try Prawn Bisque. If you plan ahead and remember to freeze prawn/shrimp heads and shells from other recipes, this rich, sophisticated soup is almost free to make.

SOUPE DE POISSONS

PREPARATION TIME 30 minutes, plus making the stock, croûtes and rouille

COOKING TIME 1 hour

3 tbsp olive oil

2 onions, sliced

4 garlic cloves, chopped

4 large tomatoes, chopped

6 tbsp long-grain white rice

900g/2lb mixed fish, such as grey mullet, haddock and monkfish, heads removed, gutted, scaled and trimmed but not boned

250g/9oz large raw prawns/shrimp, peeled and deveined, with the heads and shells reserved

4 tbsp dry white wine

1.25l/44fl oz/5½ cups Fish Stock (see page 12) or ready-made stock

1 bouquet garni made with 1 piece of celery stalk with its leaves, 1 bay leaf and several parsley and thyme sprigs tied together

1 long strip of orange zest, all bitter white pith removed

a pinch of saffron threads

3 tbsp tomato purée/paste

salt and freshly ground black pepper

TO SERVE

1 recipe quantity Croûtes (see page 17), hot

40g/1½oz/⅓ cup grated Gruyère cheese

1 recipe quantity Rouille (see page 18)

Heat the oil in a large saucepan over a medium heat. Add the onions and fry, stirring occasionally, for 3–5 minutes until softened but not coloured. Add the garlic and tomatoes and fry for 3 minutes, then add the rice, fish and prawns/shrimp, including the heads and shells. Stir in the wine and cook for 30 seconds–1 minute until evaporated. Add the stock and season with salt and pepper.

Cover and bring to the boil, then skim. Stir in the bouquet garni, orange zest, saffron and tomato purée/paste. Reduce the heat and simmer, covered, for 30–45 minutes until the fish comes off the bones and is starting to fall apart.

Discard the bouquet garni and blend the soup, including the bones and prawn/shrimp trimmings. Work the soup through a sieve into a bowl, pressing down with a spoon to extract as much flavour as possible. Rub back and forth with a spoon and scrape the bottom of the sieve. Return the soup to the rinsed-out pan and reheat. Adjust the salt and pepper, if necessary.

Divide the croûtes into bowls and top with the cheese. Ladle the soup into the bowls and serve immediately with the rouille for stirring in at the table.

BOUILLABAISSE

PREPARATION TIME 30 minutes, plus making the stock, croûtes and rouille

COOKING TIME 40 minutes

2 tbsp olive oil

1 fennel bulb, quartered and thinly sliced

1 leek, thinly sliced and rinsed

1 onion, chopped

4 garlic cloves, chopped

4 tbsp aniseed-flavoured spirit

1.25l/44fl oz/5½ cups Fish Stock (see page 12)

500ml/18fl oz/2¼ cups passata (Italian sieved tomatoes)

2 large pinches of saffron threads

12 live mussels, scrubbed, with 'beards' removed and soaked in cold water

900g/2lb mixed fish, such as sea bass, halibut, or red or grey mullet, heads removed, gutted and scaled and trimmed as necessary, boned and cut into large chunks

500g/1lb 2oz large raw prawns/shrimp, peeled and deveined

salt and freshly ground black pepper

2 recipe quantities Croûtes (see page 17), to serve

1½ recipe quantities Rouille (see page 18), to serve

Heat the oil in a saucepan over a medium heat. Add the fennel, leek and onion and fry, stirring, for 2 minutes. Add the garlic and fry for 1–3 minutes until the onion is softened. Add the spirit and cook for 2–4 minutes until almost evaporated, then add the stock, passata and saffron and season with salt and pepper. Cover and bring to the boil. Reduce the heat and simmer for 10 minutes.

Meanwhile, calculate the cooking time for the fish at 10 minutes per 2.5cm/1in of thickness. Discard any mussels with broken shells or open ones that do not close when tapped. Add the mussels to the pan and cook, covered, for 3–5 minutes, shaking the pan frequently, until all the shells open. Remove the mussels from the pan and set aside. Discard any closed mussels.

Add the fish to the pan and simmer for the calculated time until all the fish is cooked through and flakes easily. If necessary, add the fish in stages, starting with the thickest pieces. Three minutes before the end of the calculated cooking time, add the prawns/shrimp and cook until they curl and turn pink. Return the mussels in their shells to the pan and adjust the salt and pepper, if necessary. Serve with croûtes spread with rouille on the side.

AEGEAN RED MULLET SOUP

PREPARATION TIME 20 minutes, plus preparing the tomatoes

COOKING TIME 30 minutes

1½ tbsp olive oil

3 garlic cloves, finely chopped

1 leek, halved lengthways, sliced and rinsed

1 carrot, peeled and finely chopped

1 celery stalk, finely chopped

1 fennel bulb, thinly sliced

1 tbsp aniseed-flavoured spirit, such as Pernod

450g/1lb red mullet, heads and tails removed, gutted, scaled, rinsed and cut into serving pieces on the bone

2 large tomatoes, grated (see page 10)

1 bay leaf

2 tbsp orange juice

1 tbsp tomato purée/paste

grated zest of 1 orange

a pinch of saffron threads

a small pinch of dried chilli/hot pepper flakes

2 tbsp chopped parsley leaves

salt and freshly ground black pepper

Heat the oil in a saucepan over a medium heat. Stir in the garlic, leek, carrot, celery and fennel, then reduce the heat to low and cook, covered, for 8–10 minutes until softened but not coloured. Add the aniseed spirit, increase the heat to high and cook for 30 seconds–1 minute until evaporated.

Add the fish and 1.25l/44fl oz/5½ cups water and season with salt and pepper. Cover and bring to just below the boil, then skim. Stir in the tomatoes, bay leaf, orange juice, tomato purée/paste, orange zest, saffron and chilli/hot pepper flakes. Reduce the heat and simmer, covered, for 8–10 minutes until the fish flakes easily. Stir in the parsley and adjust the salt and pepper, if necessary, then serve.

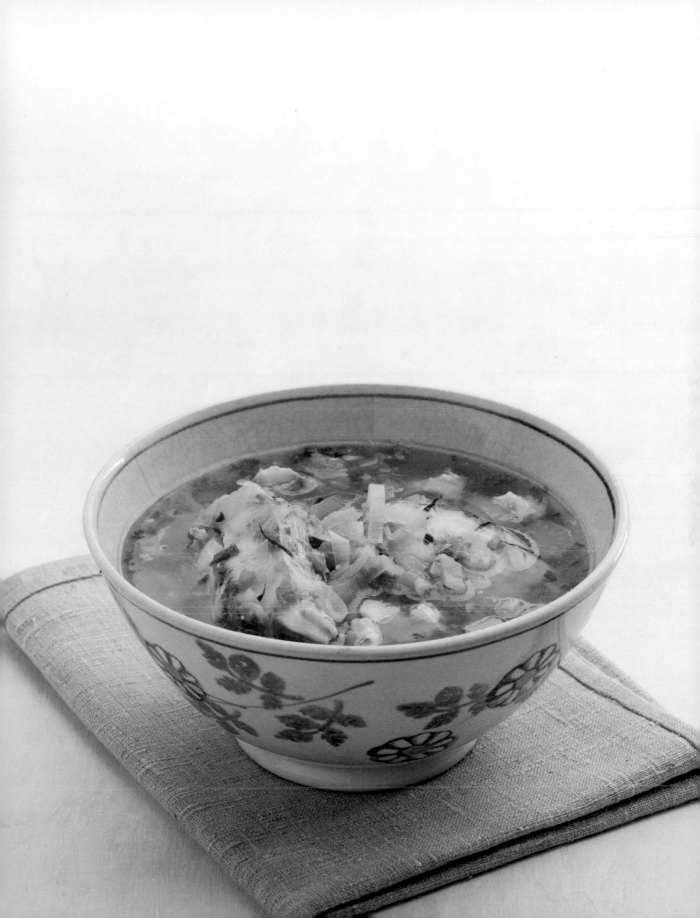

MEDITERRANEAN SWORDFISH SOUP

PREPARATION TIME 15 minutes, plus making the stock

COOKING TIME 40 minutes

3 tbsp olive oil

1 celery stalk, very finely chopped

1 onion, very finely chopped

2 large garlic cloves, crushed

1 can (400g/14oz) chopped tomatoes

240ml/8fl oz/1 cup dry white wine

1 tbsp brined or salted capers, rinsed

1.25l/44fl oz/5½ cups Fish Stock (see page 12) or ready-made stock

2 tbsp lemon juice

1 tsp dried oregano leaves

1 tsp dried thyme leaves

500g/1lb 2oz swordfish steaks

salt and freshly ground black pepper

Heat the oil in a saucepan over a medium heat. Add the celery and onion and fry, stirring occasionally, for 2 minutes. Stir in the garlic and fry for 1–3 minutes until the onion is softened but not coloured, then add the tomatoes, wine and capers and cook for 8 minutes, stirring to break up the tomatoes.

Add the stock, lemon juice, oregano and thyme and season with salt and pepper. Cover and bring to the boil, then reduce the heat and simmer for 10 minutes.

Calculate the swordfish's cooking time at 10 minutes per 2.5cm/1in of thickness, then add it to the soup and simmer, covered, for the calculated time until the swordfish flakes easily. Adjust the salt and pepper, if necessary. Remove the fish from the soup and discard any skin or bones, then flake or cut into large pieces. Divide the swordfish into bowls, ladle the soup over it and serve immediately.

SMOKED HADDOCK & SWEET POTATO CHOWDER

PREPARATION TIME 10 minutes, plus making the stock

COOKING TIME 35 minutes

2 slices of streaky bacon, rinds removed and meat chopped

½ tbsp sunflower oil

1 onion, finely chopped

2 tbsp plain white/all-purpose flour

400ml/14fl oz/1¾ cups Fish Stock (see page 12) or ready-made stock

1 large sweet potato, peeled and finely diced

400g/14oz undyed smoked haddock

240ml/8fl oz/1 cup whole milk

150ml/5fl oz/⅔ cup single/light cream

freshly grated nutmeg, to taste

cayenne pepper, to taste

salt and ground white pepper

chopped parsley leaves, to serve

Put the bacon in a saucepan over a high heat and fry for 3 minutes. Remove from the pan and set aside. Add the oil and onion to the pan and fry for 3–5 minutes until the onion is softened. Sprinkle in the flour and stir for 2 minutes, then add the stock, stirring continuously.

Add the sweet potatoes and season with white pepper. Cover and bring to the boil, then reduce the heat and simmer for 3–5 minutes until the potato is just soft.

Calculate the haddock's cooking time at 10 minutes per 2.5cm/1in of thickness. Add the fish, flesh-side down, and the milk and simmer until the flesh flakes easily. Remove the fish and set aside. Simmer until the potatoes are tender. Do not boil.

Skin and bone the fish, then flake it into the soup. Add the bacon, cream, nutmeg and cayenne pepper, then season with salt and return to just below the boil. Adjust the pepper, if necessary, and serve sprinkled with parsley.

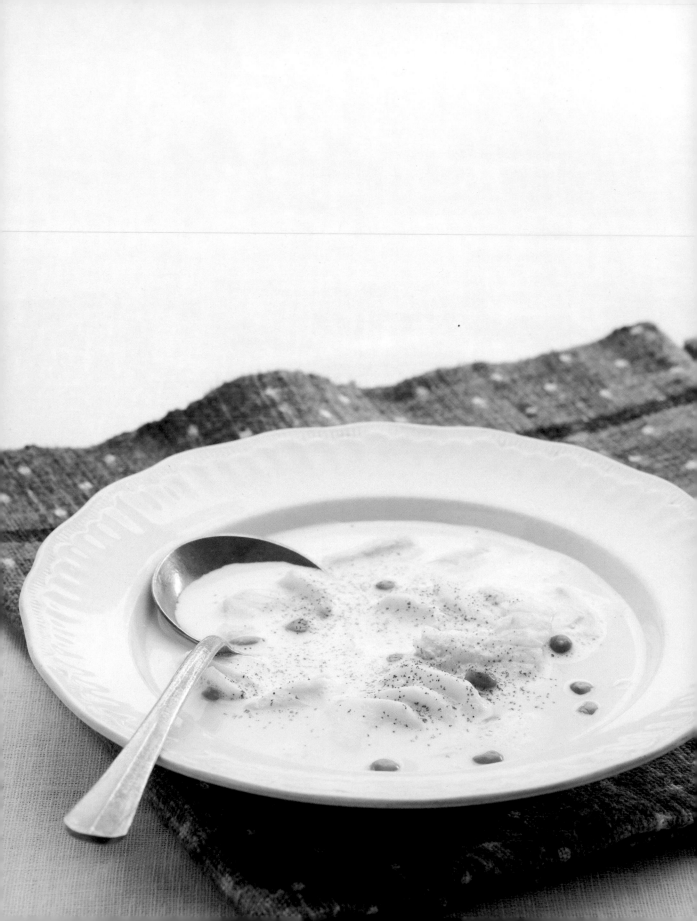

HADDOCK & PEA SOUP

PREPARATION TIME 10 minutes, plus making the stock

COOKING TIME 30 minutes

750ml/26fl oz/3¼ cups Fish Stock (see page 12) or ready-made stock

400ml/14fl oz/1¾ cups double/heavy cream

2 large garlic cloves, finely chopped

1 bay leaf

finely grated zest of ½ lemon

a pinch of ground cardamom

400g/14oz haddock fillet

200g/7oz/1¼ cups frozen peas

salt and freshly ground black pepper

smoked paprika, to serve

Put the stock, cream, garlic, bay leaf, lemon zest and cardamom in a saucepan and season with salt and pepper. Cover and bring to the boil, then reduce the heat and simmer for 10 minutes.

Calculate the haddock's cooking time at 10 minutes per 2.5cm/1in of thickness. Add the haddock and simmer, covered, for the calculated time until it is cooked through and flakes easily. Five minutes before the end of the calculated cooking time, add the peas and simmer, uncovered. Remove the haddock and set aside until cool enough to handle. Discard the bay leaf.

Bring the soup to the boil and boil for 1–2 minutes until the peas are very soft. Use a slotted spoon to transfer half the peas to a bowl. Blend the soup until smooth, and rub it through a sieve for an even smoother texture, if you like. Return the peas to the pan. Remove the skin and any small bones from the fish and flake it into large pieces into the soup. Reheat and adjust the salt and pepper, if necessary. Serve very lightly sprinkled with paprika.

CREAM OF SMOKED TROUT SOUP

PREPARATION TIME 20 minutes, plus making the stock and toasting the seeds

COOKING TIME 30 minutes

250ml/9fl oz/1 cup + 1 tbsp whole milk

2 parsley sprigs, stalks crushed

1 bay leaf

875ml/30fl oz/3¾ cups Fish Stock (see page 12) or ready-made stock

400g/14oz skinless hot-smoked trout fillets with all small bones removed

1 large onion, chopped

1 large sweet potato, peeled and diced

salt and freshly ground black pepper

TO SERVE

white sesame seeds, toasted (see page 10)

black sesame seeds

chives

Put the milk, parsley and bay leaf in a small saucepan and bring to just below the boil. Cover and set aside to infuse.

Put the stock, trout, onion and sweet potato in another saucepan and season with salt and pepper. Cover and bring to just below the boil, then reduce the heat and simmer for 10–12 minutes until the potato is tender. Remove about one-quarter of the trout and set aside.

Blend the soup until smooth. Slowly strain in enough of the infused milk to achieve the preferred consistency. Adjust the salt and pepper, if necessary, but remember the trout might be salty. Divide the soup into bowls and flake the reserved trout over it. Serve sprinkled with sesame seeds and chives.

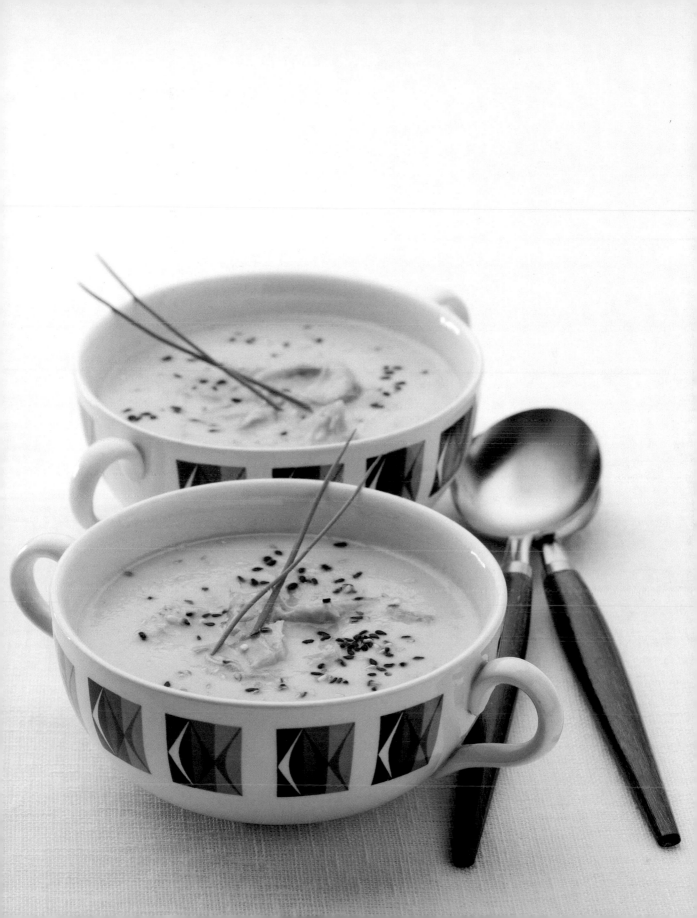

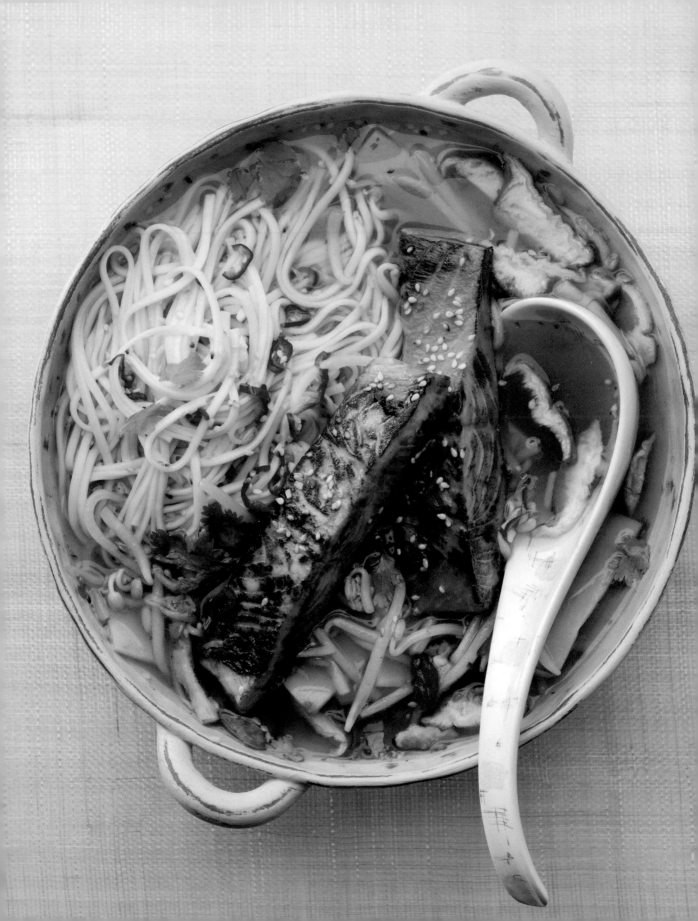

TERIYAKI SALMON RAMEN

PREPARATION TIME 15 minutes, plus making the dashi, stock and seeds
and at least 30 minutes marinating

COOKING TIME 20 minutes

750g/1lb 10oz salmon fillet, small bones removed, cut into serving portions

5 tbsp teriyaki sauce

1 tbsp sesame oil

1l/35fl oz/4½ cups Dashi (see page 13) or prepared instant dashi

1l/35fl oz/4½ cups Fish Stock (see page 12) or ready-made stock

5cm/2in piece of fresh ginger, peeled and grated

2 large garlic cloves, finely chopped

2 long red chillies, deseeded and thinly sliced

5 shiitake mushroom caps, sliced

100g/3½oz/¾ cup pickled preserved bamboo shoots

4 tsp toasted sesame oil

500g/1lb 2oz ramen noodles

1 large handful of bean sprouts, rinsed

sesame seeds, toasted (see page 10), to serve

torn coriander/cilantro leaves, to serve

Put the salmon on a plate, add the teriyaki sauce and rub it all over with your hands. Cover and chill for 30 minutes–2 hours. When ready to cook, remove from the refrigerator and heat a frying pan over a high heat until a splash of water 'dances' on the surface. Add the sesame oil to the pan and swirl around. Add the salmon, skin-side down, and cook for 3 minutes on each side or until cooked to your liking. Remove from the pan and set aside.

Meanwhile, to cook the noodles, fill a large saucepan three-quarters full of water and bring to the boil. Ramen noodles froth up so the pan needs to be very large.

Put the dashi and stock in another saucepan and bring to the boil. Reduce the heat to low, stir in the ginger, garlic, chillies, mushrooms, bamboo shoots and half the toasted sesame oil. Cover and keep warm while the noodles cook.

Add the noodles to the boiling water and cook for 4 minutes, or according to the package instructions. For the last minute of the cooking time, add the bean sprouts to the other pan to soften slightly. Drain, then divide the noodles into bowls. Divide the mushrooms, bamboo shoots and bean sprouts into the bowls, then add the salmon pieces. Ladle the soup over and serve sprinkled with the remaining toasted sesame oil, sesame seeds and coriander/cilantro.

PRAWN BISQUE

PREPARATION TIME 15 minutes, plus making the stock

COOKING TIME 50 minutes

3 tbsp butter

1 tbsp olive or hemp oil

2 shallots, finely chopped

1 carrot, peeled and chopped

1 celery stalk, thinly sliced

heads and shells from 600g/1lb 5oz raw prawns/shrimp, with 12 of the prawns/shrimp deveined and reserved (the remaining prawns/ shrimp can be frozen to use in other recipes)

2 tbsp brandy

1 can (400g/14oz) chopped tomatoes

4 tbsp dry vermouth

1 tbsp tomato purée/paste

1.4l/48fl oz/6 cups Fish Stock (see page 12) or ready-made stock

6 tbsp long-grain white rice

1 bay leaf

a pinch of dried chilli/hot pepper flakes, or to taste

½ tbsp salt, plus extra to season

1–2 tbsp lemon juice, to taste

1 tbsp chopped dill

freshly ground black pepper

lemon wedges, to serve

Melt 2 tablespoons of the butter with the oil in a saucepan over a medium heat. Add the shallots, carrot and celery and fry, stirring occasionally, for 8–10 minutes until the shallots are light golden brown. Add the prawn/shrimp shells and heads and pound them into the vegetables with a wooden spoon. Add the brandy, cook for 2–4 minutes until evaporated, then add the tomatoes, vermouth and tomato purée/paste. Bring to the boil and boil for 1–2 minutes, then add the stock, rice and bay leaf, cover and return to the boil. Skim, add the chilli/hot pepper flakes and season with salt and pepper. Reduce the heat and simmer, covered, for 15–18 minutes until the rice is tender.

Meanwhile, bring a small pan of water to the boil and add the salt. Reduce the heat, add the prawns/ shrimp and simmer for 2–3 minutes until they turn pink. Drain, cut in half lengthways and set aside.

Blend the soup until smooth, then work it through a sieve into a bowl, rubbing back and forth with a spoon and scraping the bottom of the sieve. Return the soup to the rinsed-out pan, add the lemon juice and reheat.

Melt the remaining butter in the small pan. Add the prawns/shrimp and dill and toss together just to warm through. Do not overcook. Adjust the salt and pepper and add extra lemon juice, if necessary. Divide the prawns/shrimp into bowls, ladle the soup over them and serve with lemon wedges.

PRAWN LAKSA

PREPARATION TIME 20 minutes, plus making the stock
COOKING TIME 50 minutes

500ml/18fl oz/2¼ cups Fish Stock (see page 12) or ready-made stock

1kg/2¼lb large raw prawns/shrimp, peeled and deveined, with heads and shells reserved

½ tsp salt

1 large handful of bean sprouts

12 coriander/cilantro sprigs, leaves and stalks coarsely chopped, plus extra chopped leaves to serve

5 large garlic cloves, chopped

1 bird's-eye chilli, deseeded (optional) and chopped

1 lemongrass stick, chopped, with outer leaves removed

4cm/1½in piece of fresh ginger, peeled and chopped

2 tbsp shrimp paste

½ tsp turmeric

4 tbsp groundnut/peanut or sunflower oil

1l/35fl oz/4½ cups coconut milk

1 tbsp fish sauce, or to taste

1 tbsp lime juice, or to taste

250g/9oz medium ready-to-eat rice noodles

Put the stock, prawn/shrimp heads and shells and salt in a saucepan. Cover and bring to the boil, then reduce the heat and simmer for 10 minutes. Put the bean sprouts in a bowl, cover with cold water and set aside.

Meanwhile, to make the laksa paste, put the coriander/cilantro, garlic, chilli, lemongrass, ginger, shrimp paste and turmeric in a mini food processor and blend until a paste forms. Add 3 tablespoons of the oil and blend again, then set aside.

Strain the stock through a muslin-lined/cheesecloth-lined sieve and set aside. Heat the remaining oil in a large saucepan over a high heat. Add the paste and stir-fry for 1–2 minutes until fragrant. Watch closely so it doesn't burn and add a little of the simmering stock if necessary. Stir in the stock, coconut milk, fish sauce and lime juice and bring to the boil, stirring. Cover, reduce the heat to low and simmer for 20 minutes.

Add the prawns/shrimp and simmer for 2–3 minutes until they curl and turn pink. Drain the bean sprouts and add them and the noodles to the soup and cook for 30 seconds to warm through. Adjust the fish sauce and lime juice, if necessary. Serve sprinkled with coriander/cilantro.

PRAWN BALL SOUP

PREPARATION TIME 25 minutes, plus making the dashi and at least 15 minutes chilling
COOKING TIME 25 minutes

400g/14oz raw prawns/shrimp, peeled, deveined and finely chopped, with heads and shells reserved

1 small egg, beaten

1 tbsp cornflour/cornstarch

1 recipe quantity Dashi (see page 13) or 1.25l/44fl oz/5½ cups prepared instant dashi

2 tsp salt

1 tsp sesame oil

coriander/cilantro leaves or baby shiso leaves, to serve

very finely julienned zest of 1 lemon, to serve

Put the prawns/shrimp in a bowl and use your fingers to gradually incorporate the egg to make a sticky paste – you might not need all the egg. Sprinkle in the cornflour/cornstarch, mix again and shape into a loose ball. 'Throw' this ball against the inside of the bowl several times to soften the mixture and help it stick together more, then cover and chill for at least 15 minutes.

Meanwhile, put the dashi and prawn/shrimp heads and shells in a saucepan. Cover and bring to just below the boil, then reduce the heat to very low (use a heat diffuser if you have one) and simmer while you prepare the prawn balls. Do not boil.

Divide the salt between two saucepans of water, cover and bring each to the boil. Put the prawn ball on a plate and sprinkle with the sesame oil, letting the excess slide onto the plate – this makes it easier to roll the mixture. Divide the mixture into 36 portions.

Roll the portions into balls. Divide them between the two pans of slowly boiling water and boil gently for 1½–2 minutes until they float to the surface. Remove from the water and set aside.

Strain the dashi into one of the rinsed-out pans and return to just below the boil. Immediately reduce the heat to low, add the prawn balls and warm through. Divide the balls into bowls, ladle the soup over them and serve topped with coriander/cilantro and lemon zest.

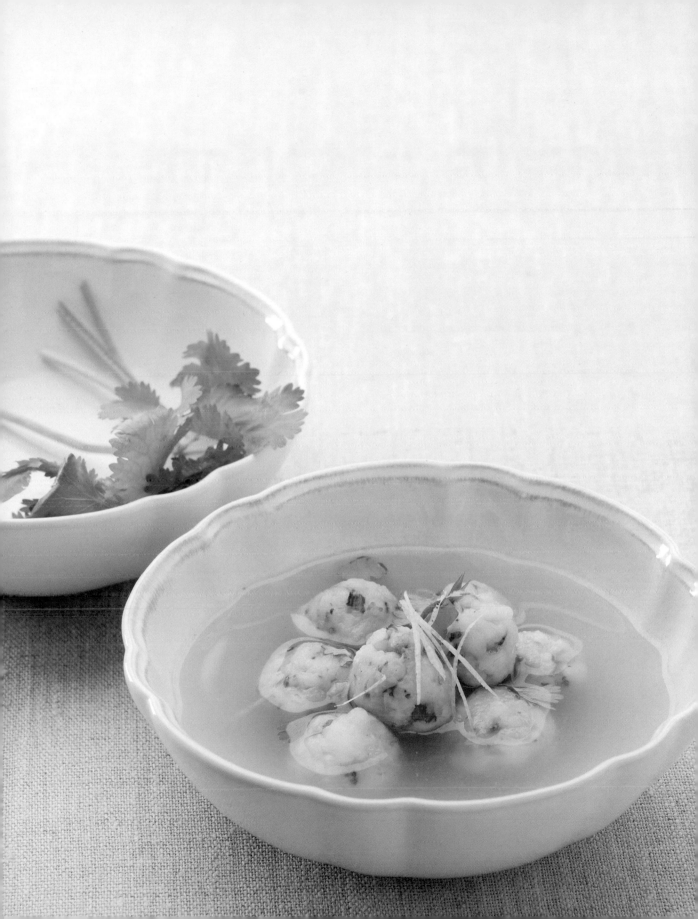

SCANDINAVIAN SALMON & PRAWN SOUP

PREPARATION TIME 20 minutes, plus making the stock and preparing the tomato
COOKING TIME 30 minutes

1 tbsp butter

1 tbsp sunflower oil

½ leek, halved lengthways, thinly sliced and rinsed

1 floury/russet potato, peeled and chopped

1 large ripe tomato, peeled (see page 10), deseeded and finely chopped

400g/14oz skinless salmon fillet, any small bones removed

1l/35fl oz/4½ cups Fish Stock (see page 12) or ready-made stock

1 bay leaf

a pinch of cayenne pepper

a pinch of ground cardamom

250g/9oz medium raw prawns/shrimp, peeled and deveined

3 tbsp chopped dill

salt and freshly ground black pepper

Melt the butter with the oil in a saucepan over a medium heat. Stir in the leek, potato and tomato, reduce the heat to low and cook, covered, for 10 minutes until the vegetables are softened but not coloured. Meanwhile, calculate the salmon's cooking time at 10 minutes per 2.5cm/1in of thickness.

Add the stock, bay leaf, cayenne pepper and cardamom and season with salt and pepper. Cover and bring to the boil. Reduce the heat to low, add the salmon and simmer, covered, for 3 minutes less than the calculated time.

Stir in the prawns/shrimp and simmer for 2–3 minutes until they turn pink and curl and the salmon flakes easily. If the prawns/shrimp are cooked before the salmon remove them from the pan and set aside. Discard the bay leaf, then stir in the dill and return the prawns/shrimp, if necessary. Adjust the salt and pepper, if necessary, and serve.

THAI HOT-AND-SOUR SOUP WITH PRAWNS

PREPARATION TIME 20 minutes

COOKING TIME 20 minutes

4 lemongrass sticks, cut into 3 pieces and lightly crushed, with outer leaves removed

4 coriander/cilantro sprigs, including roots and stalks, cut in half, plus extra chopped leaves to serve

6 kaffir lime leaves, torn

12 button mushrooms, sliced

1 tsp salt

24 large raw prawns/shrimp, peeled and deveined

3 tbsp lime juice

2 tbsp fish sauce

1–2 bird's-eye chillies, deseeded (optional) and diagonally sliced

lime wedges, to serve

Bring 1.25l/44fl oz/5½ cups water to the boil in a saucepan. Add the lemongrass, coriander/cilantro, lime leaves, mushrooms and salt and boil, covered, for 5 minutes.

Reduce the heat to low, add the prawns/shrimp and simmer for 2–3 minutes until they turn pink and curl. Immediately stir in the lime juice, fish sauce and chillies. Discard the lemongrass and coriander/cilantro. Serve sprinkled with coriander/cilantro leaves and with lime wedges for squeezing over.

CARIBBEAN CALLALOO

PREPARATION TIME 15 minutes, plus making the stock

COOKING TIME 40 minutes

1 tbsp butter

2 tbsp sunflower or groundnut/peanut oil

1 large onion, chopped

2 garlic cloves, finely chopped

600g/1lb 5oz callaloo greens or spinach, chopped

1.25l/44fl oz/5½ cups Chicken Stock (see page 12)

800ml/28fl oz/3½ cups coconut milk

400g/14oz floury potatoes, peeled and chopped

350g/12oz shelled white crabmeat

salt and freshly ground black pepper

paprika and hot pepper sauce, to serve

Melt the butter with the oil in a saucepan over a medium heat. Add the onion and fry, stirring, for 2 minutes. Stir in the garlic and fry for 1–3 minutes until the onion is softened. Add the greens and stir for 5 minutes until they wilt, then remove them from the pan and set aside. Add the stock, coconut milk and potatoes to the pan and season with salt and pepper. Cover and bring to the boil, then reduce the heat and simmer, partially covered, for 10–12 minutes until the potatoes are tender.

Return the greens to the pan and simmer for 5–8 minutes until they are tender. Stir in the crabmeat and simmer for 3 minutes until cooked. Adjust the seasoning, if necessary, and serve sprinkled with paprika and with hot pepper sauce on the side.

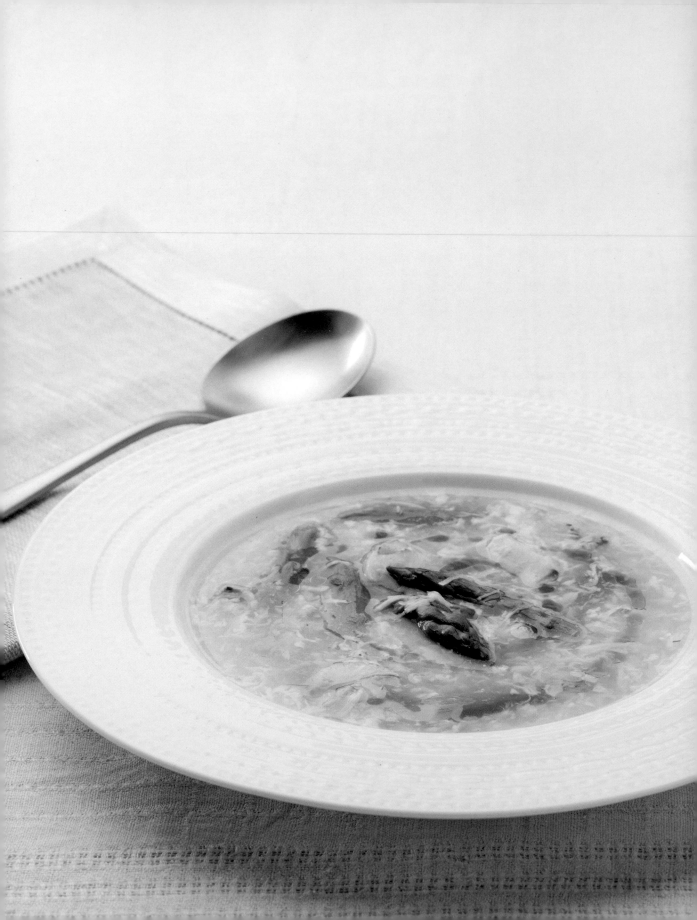

CRAB & ASPARAGUS SOUP

PREPARATION TIME 10 minutes, plus making the stock

COOKING TIME 25 minutes

2 tbsp arrowroot

1.25l/44fl oz/5½ cups Chicken Stock (see page 12) or ready-made stock

1 tbsp fish sauce

½ tsp salt, plus extra to season

350g/12oz/2½ cups trimmed asparagus cut into bite-size pieces, with the tips reserved

1 egg

175g/6oz shelled white crabmeat, thawed if frozen, picked over and flaked

ground white pepper

toasted sesame oil, to drizzle

Put the arrowroot and 2 tablespoons of the stock in a bowl and mix until smooth, then set aside. Put the remaining stock in a saucepan over a medium heat and bring to a simmer. Pour the arrowroot mixture into the stock, whisking continuously, then bring to just below the boil, stirring. Stir in the fish sauce and salt, reduce the heat and simmer for 2–3 minutes, stirring, until the soup thickens slightly.

Add the asparagus stalks and simmer for 3 minutes, then add the asparagus tips and simmer for another 3–5 minutes until all the asparagus is tender but still has a little bite. Return the soup to the boil.

Meanwhile, beat the egg in a heatproof bowl, add a ladleful of the hot stock and whisk together.

Remove the pan from the heat and pour the egg mixture in a steady stream into the middle of the soup with one hand while beating continuously in a circular motion with a chopstick or fork in the other hand until long, thin strands of egg form. Stir in the crab and cook over a very low heat for 2–3 minutes until the crabmeat is heated through. Season with salt and white pepper and serve immediately drizzled with sesame oil.

NEW ENGLAND CLAM CHOWDER

PREPARATION TIME 20 minutes

COOKING TIME 50 minutes

55g/2oz/⅓ cup diced unsmoked streaky bacon

2 tbsp butter

2 celery stalks, finely chopped

2 onions, finely chopped

1 tbsp plain white/all-purpose flour

600ml/20fl oz/2½ cups whole milk

400g/14oz floury/russet potatoes, peeled and diced

48 live littleneck clams, rinsed and soaked in cold water to cover

2 tsp dried thyme leaves

600ml/20fl oz/2½ cups single/light cream

salt and freshly ground black pepper

cayenne pepper, to serve

oyster crackers, to serve (optional)

Put the bacon in a saucepan over a high heat and fry, stirring, for 5–8 minutes until it crisps and gives off its fat. Remove it from the pan and set aside.

Melt the butter in the fat remaining in the pan. Stir in the celery and onions, cover, reduce the heat to low and cook for 8–10 minutes until softened but not coloured. Increase the heat to medium, sprinkle in the flour and stir for 2 minutes, then slowly add the milk, stirring continuously to prevent lumps from forming. Add the potatoes and season with salt and pepper. Bring to just below the boil, cover and simmer for 15–20 minutes until the potatoes are tender.

Meanwhile, discard any clams with broken shells or open ones that do not close when tapped. Shuck the clams over a bowl to catch the juices. Discard the shells and chop the clams, then stir them with the juices, thyme and bacon into the soup.

Cover and simmer for 1 minute. Stir in the cream and simmer for 1–2 minutes until the clams are cooked through. Adjust the salt and pepper, if necessary, then serve sprinkled with cayenne pepper and with oyster crackers on the side, if you like.

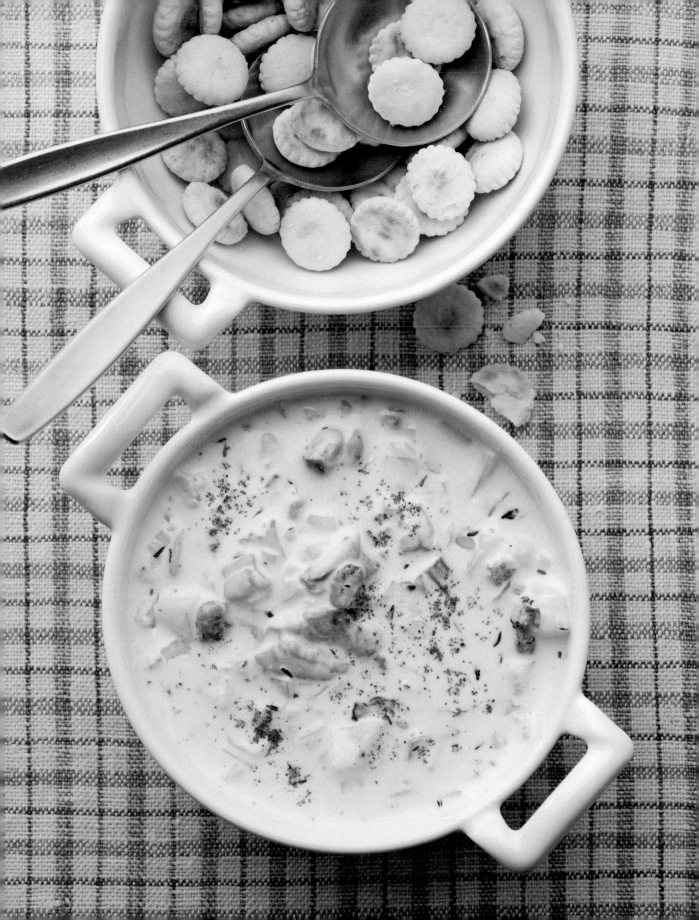

SAFFRON-SCENTED MUSSEL SOUP

PREPARATION TIME 30 minutes, plus making the stock

COOKING TIME 45 minutes

1l/35fl oz/4½ cups Fish Stock (see page 12) or ready-made stock

a large pinch of saffron threads

1.25kg/2¾lb live mussels, scrubbed, with 'beards' removed and soaked in cold water to cover

3 tbsp olive or hemp oil

2 large garlic cloves, finely chopped

1 carrot, peeled and diced

1 celery stalk, thinly sliced

1 fennel bulb, sliced

1 leek, halved lengthways, sliced and rinsed

150ml/5fl oz/⅔ cup dry white wine

1 bouquet garni made with 1 bay leaf, 1 parsley sprig, 1 rosemary sprig and 1 thyme sprig tied together

lemon juice, to taste

salt and freshly ground black pepper

Put the stock and saffron in a saucepan, cover and bring to the boil, then remove from the heat and set aside, covered, for the flavours to blend.

Discard any cracked mussels or open ones that do not close when tapped. Put the mussels and 240ml/8fl oz/1 cup water in another saucepan and cook, covered, over a medium heat for 5–8 minutes, shaking the pan frequently, until they all open. Strain the cooking liquid through a muslin-lined/cheesecloth-lined sieve, then add it to the saffron-flavoured stock. Set the mussels aside until cool enough to handle, then discard any that are still closed. Remove the mussels from the shells and set aside.

Meanwhile, heat the oil in the rinsed-out pan over a medium heat. Add the garlic, carrot, celery, fennel and leek and fry, stirring, for 2 minutes. Reduce the heat to low and cook, covered, for 8–10 minutes, stirring occasionally, until all the vegetables are softened but not coloured. Add the stock, white wine and bouquet garni and season with salt. Cover and bring to the boil, then reduce the heat and simmer for 5 minutes.

Discard the bouquet garni and stir the mussels into the soup to warm through – take care not to overcook or they will toughen. Adjust the salt and pepper and add lemon juice, if necessary, then serve.

ELEGANT JAPANESE SCALLOP SOUP

PREPARATION TIME 5 minutes, plus making the dashi

COOKING TIME 10 minutes

1 recipe quantity Dashi (see page 13) or 1.25l/ 44fl oz/5½ cups prepared instant dashi

4 tsp soy sauce or tamari soy sauce

2 tsp sake or dry sherry

½ tsp salt, plus extra to season

1 large shelled queen scallop for each bowl, coral removed and reserved and each scallop cut into 3 equal horizontal slices

shiso or coriander/cilantro leaves, to serve

grated yuzu or lemon zest, to serve

Put the dashi, soy sauce, sake and salt in a saucepan. Cover and bring to just below the boil. Reduce the heat and simmer for 1 minute. Adjust the salt, if necessary.

Arrange the scallop slices and coral in bowls and ladle the soup over them. Add a shiso leaf to each, sprinkle with yuzu zest and serve.

MACKEREL IN CHILLI-LIME BROTH

PREPARATION TIME 10 minutes, plus making the stock

COOKING TIME 25 minutes

1.4l/48fl oz/6 cups Fish Stock (see page 12) or ready-made stock

6 kaffir lime leaves, lightly crushed

2.5cm/1in piece of fresh ginger, peeled and grated

1 red chilli, deseeded and sliced

2 tbsp light soy sauce or tamari soy sauce

1 tbsp fish sauce

400g/14oz mackerel fillets

finely grated zest of 1 lime

freshly ground black pepper

shiso leaves or coriander/cilantro leaves, to serve

lime wedges, to serve

Put the stock, lime leaves, ginger, chilli, soy sauce and fish sauce in a saucepan. Cover and bring to the boil, then reduce the heat and simmer for 10 minutes. Add the mackerel and simmer, covered, for 2–3 minutes until the fillets flake easily. Remove the mackerel from the pan and remove the skin.

Flake the fish into the soup, add the lime zest and season with pepper. Serve topped with shiso leaves and with lime wedges for squeezing over.

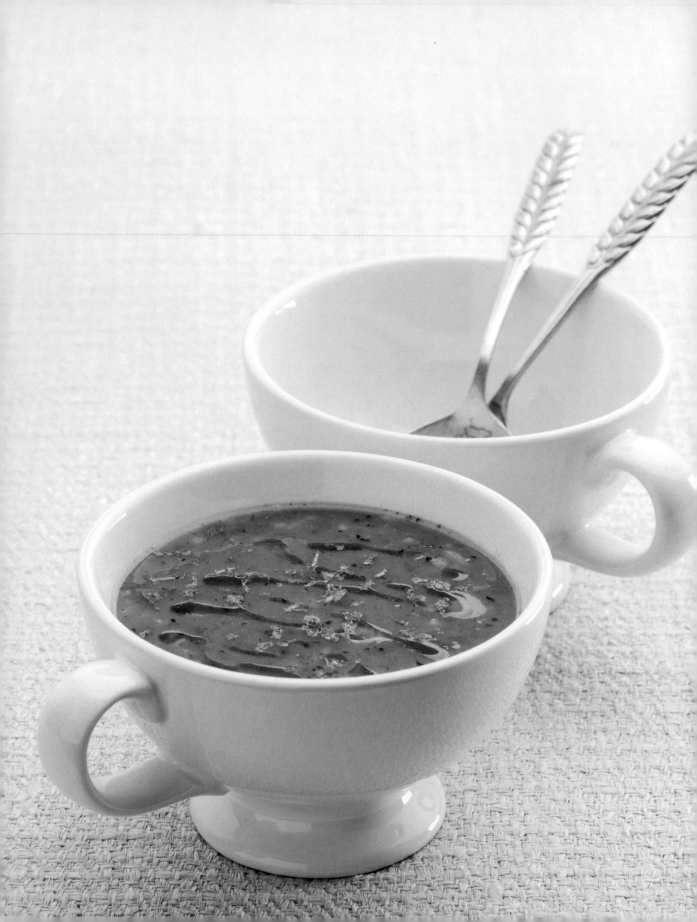

VEGETABLE
& GRAIN SOUPS

This chapter is a cornucopia of recipes that celebrate the seasons. Brighten up the cold, bleak winter months with hearty, colourful blends of carrot, pumpkin and beetroot/beets. Usher in spring with the intense green colour and fresh flavours of peas, spinach and sorrel. Then, when warmer summer temperatures make you long for lighter choices, enjoy the Mediterranean influences of tomatoes, peppers and herbs.

You'll also find four seasonal farmers' market soups, one for each season, designed to make the most of produce at its best – and least expensive. Once you're in the habit of regularly making Vegetable Stock (page 12) you'll have the foundation to make a soup with any ingredients you find in the market.

None of the soups in this chapter contain meat, but a couple of recipes do suggest using meat stock for a rich, savoury base flavour. This can easily be substituted with homemade vegetable stock if you would prefer to keep your meal meat-free. Similarly, though many of the recipes contain dairy products, if you are following a vegan diet there are still plenty of choices. Arame & Tofu Soup is a tempting option when made with vegetarian dashi, and Edamame & Pumpkin Soup is also vegan-friendly. (Vegans can also enjoy the Bloody Mary Party Soup and Minted Pea Soup in the Chilled Soups chapter.)

BROCCOLI & PARSLEY SOUP

PREPARATION TIME 15 minutes, plus making the stock and pumpkin seeds

COOKING TIME 30 minutes

1 tbsp sunflower oil

2 shallots, chopped

2 large garlic cloves, finely chopped

1l/35fl oz/4½ cups Vegetable Stock (see page 12) or ready-made stock

350g/12oz broccoli, cut into florets and the stalks sliced

1 bunch of curly-leaf parsley, about 30g/1oz, leaves and stems chopped

a pinch of dried chilli/hot pepper flakes, or to taste

1 Parmesan or other cheese rind, about 7.5 x 5cm/3 x 2in (see page 9; optional)

salt and freshly ground black pepper

Roasted Pumpkin Seeds (see page 19), to serve

chopped chives, to serve (optional)

Heat the oil in a saucepan over a medium heat. Add the shallots and fry, stirring occasionally, for 2 minutes. Stir in the garlic and fry for another 1–3 minutes until the shallots are softened but not coloured.

Add the stock, broccoli, parsley, chilli/hot pepper flakes and cheese rind, if using, and season with salt and pepper, but remember the rind will be salty, if you are using it, so you might not need to add much salt. Cover and bring to the boil, then reduce the heat and simmer for 15–20 minutes until the broccoli stalks are very tender.

Discard the cheese rind, if used. Blend the soup, then adjust the salt and pepper, if necessary. Serve sprinkled with the seeds and chives, if you like.

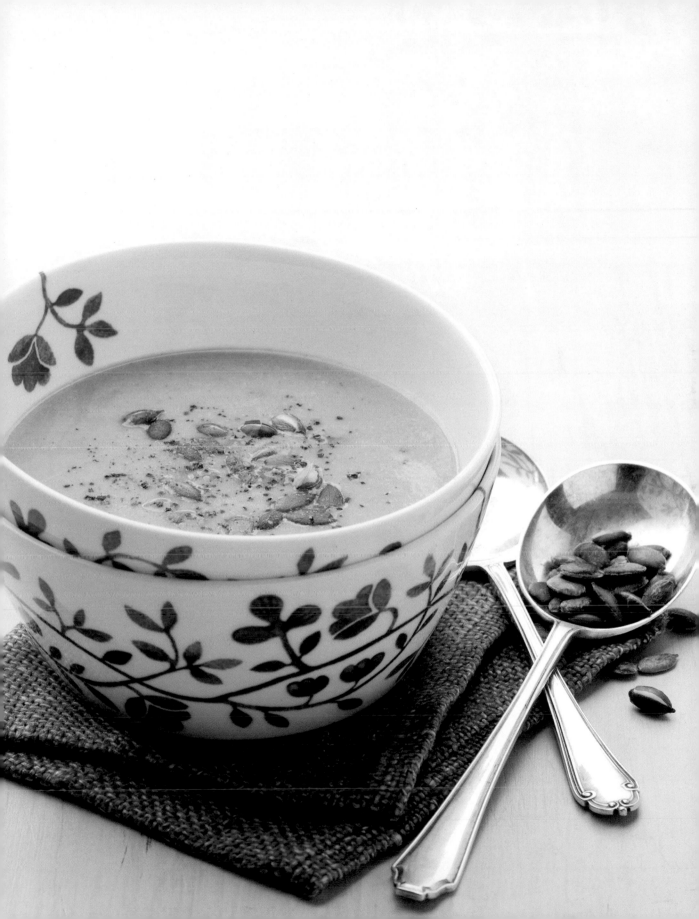

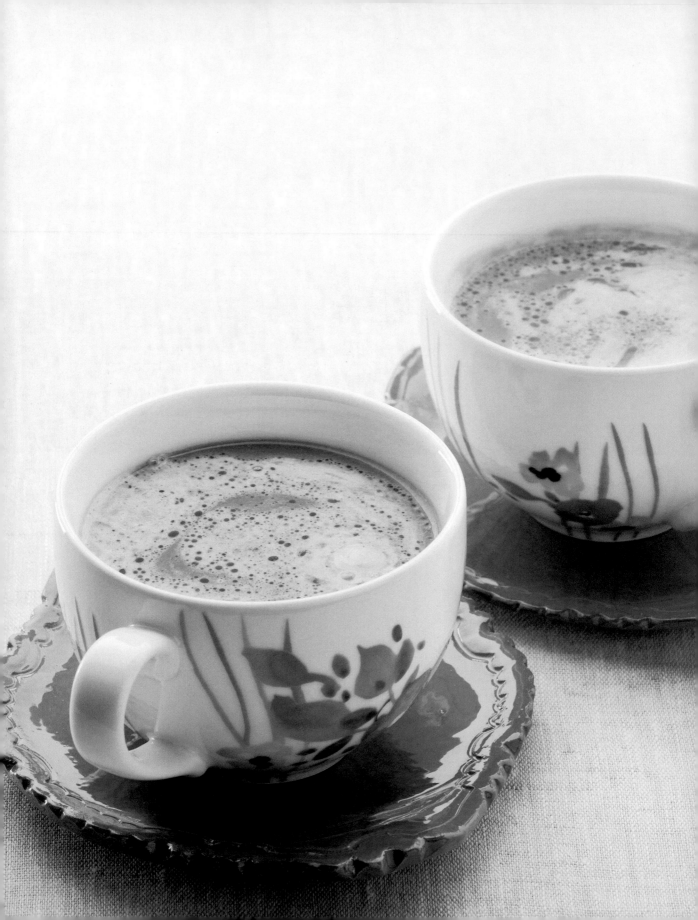

SPRING SORREL & SPINACH SOUP WITH EGG BUTTERBALLS

PREPARATION TIME 25 minutes, plus making the stock and cooking the eggs

COOKING TIME 40 minutes

2 tbsp butter

1 tbsp olive or hemp oil

1 large onion, chopped

4 large garlic cloves, chopped

100g/3½oz/1½ cups young sorrel leaves, stalks crushed

2 handfuls of baby spinach leaves

1.25l/44fl oz/5½ cups Vegetable Stock (see page 12) or ready-made stock

2 tbsp chopped parsley leaves

salt and freshly ground black pepper

EGG BUTTERBALLS

100g/3½oz/7 tbsp butter, at room temperature

2 large/extra-large hard-boiled egg yolks, chopped

a pinch of turmeric

a pinch of cayenne pepper (optional)

Melt the butter with the oil in a saucepan over a medium heat. Add the onion and garlic, reduce the heat to low and cook, covered, for 10–12 minutes until very tender and just starting to turn golden. Add the sorrel and spinach and stir for 3–5 minutes until wilted. Add the stock and parsley and season with salt and pepper.

Bring to the boil, partially covered. Reduce the heat and simmer, partially covered, for 10–15 minutes until the leaves are very tender.

Meanwhile, make the butterballs. Put the butter, egg yolks, turmeric and cayenne pepper, if using, in a bowl and beat together. Season with salt and pepper, then divide the mixture into 12 equal portions and roll into balls. (The butterballs can be made up to 1 day in advance and chilled until required.)

Blend the soup until smooth, then work it through a sieve into a bowl, rubbing back and forth with a spoon and scraping the bottom of the sieve. Return to the pan, adjust the salt and pepper, if necessary, and reheat. Add the butterballs and serve.

SLOW-COOKED TOMATO & ORANGE SOUP

PREPARATION TIME 15 minutes, plus making the stock and croûtes (optional)
COOKING TIME 1¼ hours

2 tbsp butter

1 tbsp olive or hemp oil

2 celery stalks, finely chopped

2 shallots, finely chopped

2 large garlic cloves, finely chopped

750g/1lb 10oz/4¼ cups chopped juicy tomatoes

1l/35fl oz/4½ cups Vegetable Stock (see page 12) or ready-made stock

a pinch of sugar

a pinch of cayenne pepper

finely grated zest of 1 orange

2–4 tbsp orange juice

salt and freshly ground black pepper

1 recipe quantity Goats' Cheese Croûtes (see page 17), to serve (optional)

Melt the butter with the oil in a saucepan over a medium heat. Add the celery and shallots and fry, stirring occasionally, for 2 minutes. Stir in the garlic and fry for another 1–3 minutes until the shallots are softened but not coloured. Add the tomatoes and stir for 2 minutes, then stir in the stock, sugar and cayenne pepper, and season with salt and pepper. Cover and bring to the boil, then reduce the heat to low (use a heat diffuser if you have one) and simmer for 1 hour.

Strain the soup to remove the tomato seeds and skins, rubbing back and forth with a spoon and scraping the bottom of the sieve. Return the soup to the pan and blot with folded paper towels to remove the excess fat from the surface. Stir in the orange zest and 2 tablespoons of the orange juice and reheat. Adjust the salt and pepper, and add more orange juice, if you like. Serve with croûtes, if you like.

WINTER FARMERS' MARKET SOUP

PREPARATION TIME 20 minutes, plus making the stock and seeds

COOKING TIME 30 minutes

1 tbsp butter

1 tbsp olive or hemp oil

1 large carrot, peeled and diced

1 head of chicory/Belgian endive, halved lengthways and sliced

1 waxy or small red potato, peeled and diced

1 large onion, finely chopped

1 shallot, finely chopped

200g/7oz/1¼ cups peeled and diced celeriac/celery root

1.25l/44fl oz/5½ cups Vegetable Stock (see page 12) or ready-made stock

1 bouquet garni made with 1 piece of celery stalk, 1 bay leaf and several parsley and thyme sprigs tied together

4 tbsp crème fraîche or sour cream

2 tbsp chopped chives

2 spring onions/scallions, thinly sliced

salt and freshly ground black pepper

Spiced Seeds (see page 19), to serve

1 roasted red pepper in olive oil, drained and diced, to serve

Melt the butter with the oil in a saucepan over a medium heat. Add the carrot, chicory/Belgian endive, potato, onion, shallot and celeriac/celery root and fry, stirring, for 3–5 minutes until the onion is softened but not coloured. Add the stock and bouquet garni and season with salt and pepper. Cover and bring to the boil, then reduce the heat and simmer for 10–15 minutes until the vegetables are tender. Discard the bouquet garni.

Blend one-third of the soup until smooth, then return it to the pan. Add the crème fraîche, chives and spring onions/scallions and reheat, then adjust the salt and pepper, if necessary. Serve sprinkled with the seeds and red pepper.

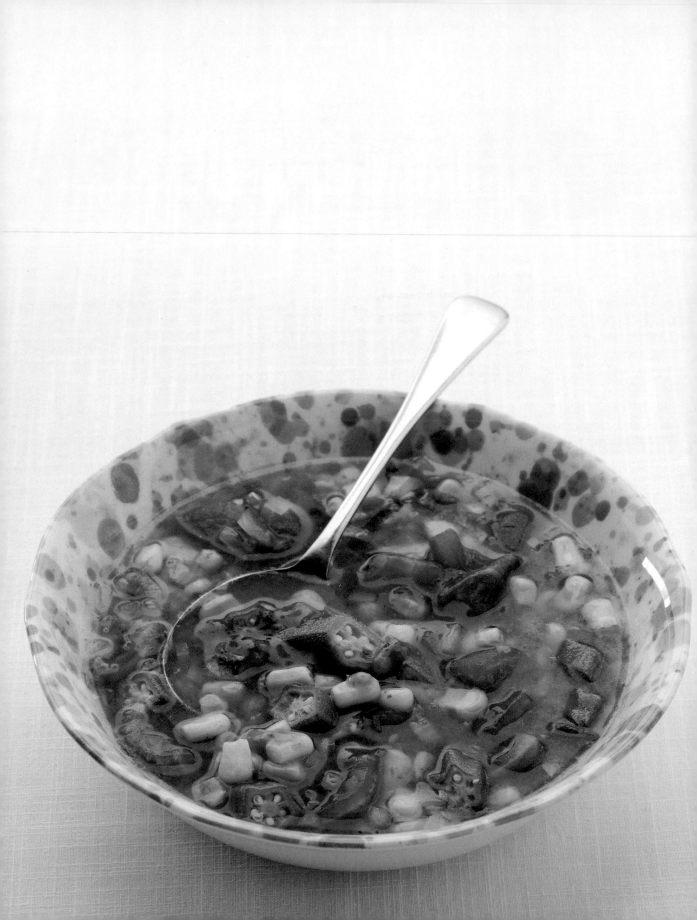

OKRA & SWEETCORN SOUP

PREPARATION TIME 15 minutes, plus 30 minutes soaking the okra,
making the stock and chilli bon-bon and preparing the tomatoes

COOKING TIME 30 minutes

100g/3½oz/1 cup sliced okra

1 tbsp white wine vinegar

½ tsp salt, plus extra to season

1 tbsp sunflower oil

1 onion, finely chopped

2 garlic cloves, chopped

1.25l/44fl oz/5½ cups Vegetable Stock
(see page 12) or ready-made stock

a pinch of dried chilli/hot pepper flakes (optional)

4 large tomatoes, peeled (see page 10),
deseeded and chopped

400g/14oz/2⅔ cups frozen sweetcorn/
corn kernels

1 tbsp tomato purée/paste

2 tbsp chopped curly parsley leaves

freshly ground black pepper

Chilli Bon-Bon (see page 19) or hot pepper
sauce, to serve (optional)

Put the okra, vinegar and salt in a large bowl. Cover with water and leave to soak for 30 minutes, then drain, rinse, drain again and set aside. This helps to reduce the okra's sliminess while it cooks.

Heat the oil in a saucepan over a medium heat. Add the onion and fry, stirring occasionally, for 2 minutes. Add the garlic and okra and fry, stirring continuously, for 3–6 minutes until the onion is softened and light golden brown. Add the stock and chilli/hot pepper flakes, if using, and season with salt and pepper. Cover and bring to the boil, then reduce the heat and simmer for 5 minutes.

Stir in the tomatoes, sweetcorn/corn and tomato purée/paste and simmer for 5–10 minutes until the okra is tender. Stir in the parsley and adjust the salt and pepper, if necessary. Serve with chilli bon-bon for adding at the table, if wished.

LEEK, SWEET POTATO & HERB SOUP

PREPARATION TIME 15 minutes, plus making the stock

COOKING TIME 15 minutes

1 small handful of chervil

1 small handful of thyme

2 tarragon sprigs

1 large handful of curly-leaf parsley, leaves finely chopped and stalks reserved and lightly crushed

1 small handful of chives, half of them chopped and kept separate

1.5l/52fl oz/6½ cups Vegetable Stock (see page 12) or ready-made stock

2 leeks, sliced in half lengthways, thinly sliced and rinsed

1 tbsp butter

1 tbsp sunflower, olive or hemp oil

280g/10oz/2 cups peeled and diced sweet potatoes

salt and freshly ground black pepper

Strip the leaves from half the chervil, thyme and tarragon sprigs and mix them together with the chopped parsley and chopped chives, then set aside.

Put the parsley stalks, whole chives and whole chervil, thyme and tarragon sprigs in a saucepan. Add the stock and half the leeks and season lightly with salt. Cover and bring to the boil, then boil, uncovered, for 10 minutes.

Meanwhile, melt the butter with the oil in a saucepan over a medium heat. Stir in the sweet potatoes and remaining leek and reduce the heat to low. Cook, covered, for 8–10 minutes, stirring occasionally, until the leek is softened but not coloured.

Strain the stock into the pan with the sweet potatoes, pressing down to extract as much flavour as possible. Bring to the boil, uncovered, then reduce the heat and simmer for 2–3 minutes until the potatoes are tender. Adjust the salt and pepper, if necessary. Just before serving, stir in the chopped herbs and simmer for no more than 30 seconds, then serve.

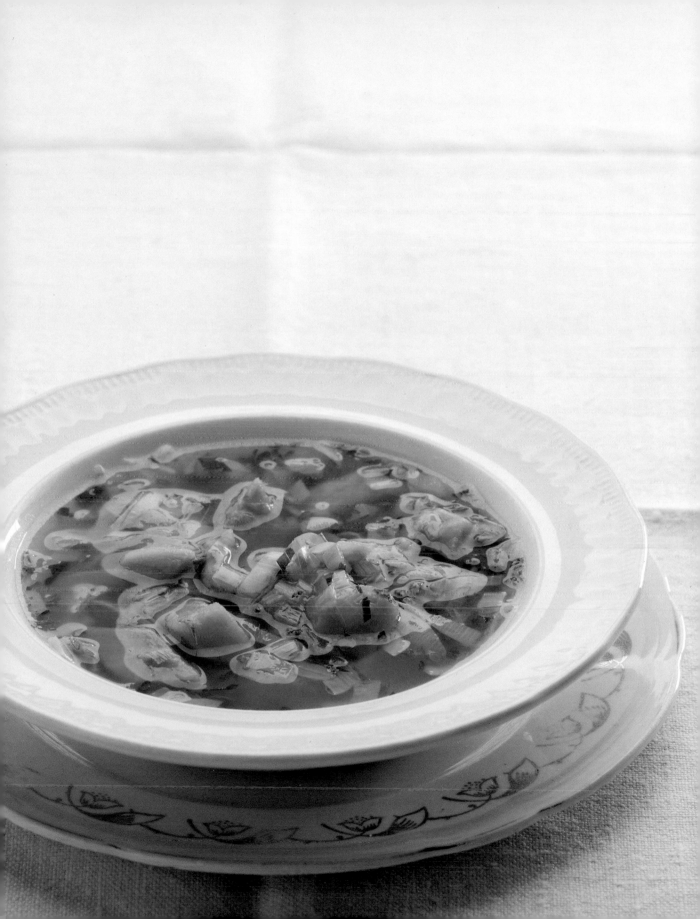

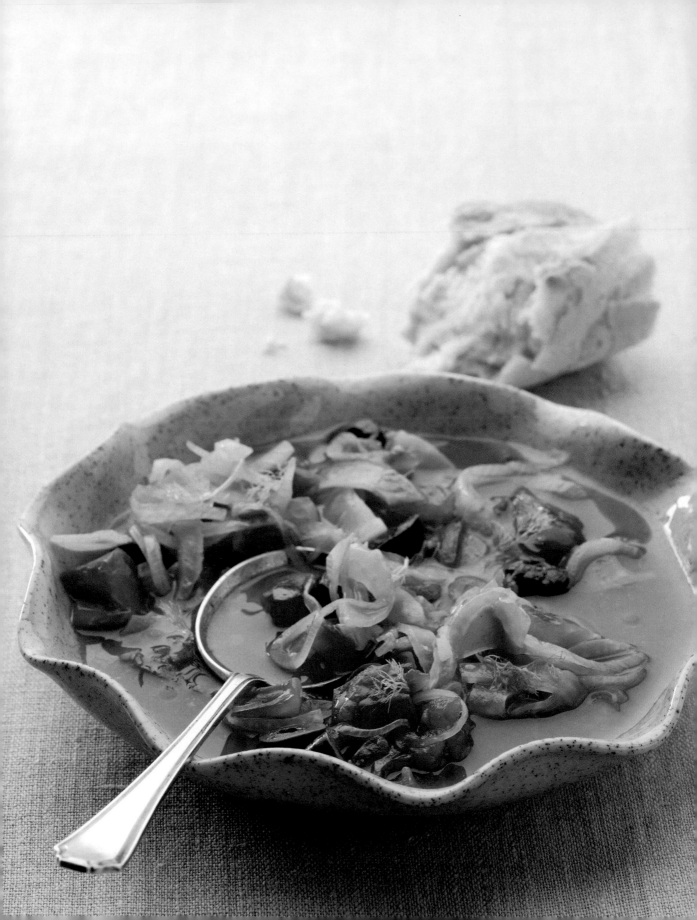

MEDITERRANEAN FENNEL SOUP

PREPARATION TIME 15 minutes, plus making the stock

COOKING TIME 45 minutes

2 tbsp garlic-flavoured olive oil

2 large fennel bulbs, sliced, with the fronds reserved

2 shallots, sliced

1 tsp fennel seeds

125ml/4fl oz/½ cup dry white wine

650g/1½lb/4 cups fresh chopped tomatoes

1 tbsp tomato purée/paste

1l/35fl oz/4½ cups Vegetable Stock (see page 12) or ready-made stock

85g/3oz/⅔ cup large pitted black olives, sliced

salt and freshly ground black pepper

French bread, to serve

Heat the oil in a large saucepan over a medium heat. Add the fennel and shallots and fry, stirring occasionally, for 3–5 minutes until the shallots are softened but not coloured. Add the fennel seeds and stir for 30 seconds. Stir in the wine, increase the heat to high and cook for 5–6 minutes until almost evaporated.

Add the tomatoes, tomato purée/paste, stock and olives and season with pepper. Do not add salt at this point because the olives will be salty. Cover and bring to the boil, then reduce the heat and simmer for 20–25 minutes. Adjust the salt and pepper, but remember salt might not be necessary. Serve sprinkled with the fennel fronds and with French bread on the side.

PARMESAN BROTH WITH PEAS & CARROTS

PREPARATION TIME 15 minutes, plus making
the stock

COOKING TIME 35 minutes

1.4l/48fl oz/6 cups Vegetable Stock
(see page 12) or ready-made stock

1 onion, peeled and quartered

1 Parmesan cheese rind, about 7.5 x 5cm/
3 x 2in (see page 9)

100g/3½oz/⅔ cup frozen peas

100g/3½oz/1 cup diced carrot, the same size
as the peas

2 Cos/romaine lettuce leaves, finely chopped

salt and freshly ground black pepper

extra-virgin olive oil, to serve

freshly grated Parmesan cheese, to serve

Put the stock, onion and cheese rind in a
saucepan, cover and bring to the boil, then
reduce the heat and simmer for 20 minutes.

Discard the onion. Return the stock to the boil,
add the peas and carrots and boil, uncovered, for
3–5 minutes until they are tender. Stir in the lettuce
and simmer for 30 seconds until wilted. Season
with salt and pepper, but remember the cheese
rind will have been salty. Discard the rind. Serve
drizzled with oil and with Parmesan cheese for
adding at the table.

ORZO PRIMAVERA SOUP

PREPARATION TIME 15 minutes, plus making
the stock

COOKING TIME 40 minutes

1.4l/48fl oz/6 cups Vegetable Stock
(see page 12) or ready-made stock

1 bouquet garni made with 1 piece of celery stalk
with its leaves, 1 rosemary sprig and several
parsley and thyme sprigs tied together

1 young carrot, diced

1 young turnip, peeled and diced

100g/3½oz/½ cup orzo

85g/3oz/¾ cup chopped green beans

80g/2¾oz/½ cup frozen peas

1 tsp finely grated lemon zest

2 tbsp chopped parsley leaves

salt and freshly ground black pepper

Put the stock and bouquet garni in a saucepan
over a high heat and season with salt and pepper.
Cover and bring to the boil, then reduce the heat
and simmer for 10 minutes.

Return the stock to the boil, add the carrot and
turnip and boil for 2 minutes. Stir in the orzo and
boil for 11 minutes, then add the green beans
and peas and boil for 4–6 minutes until the orzo
and vegetables are tender. Discard the bouquet
garni. Stir in the lemon zest and adjust the salt and
pepper, if necessary. Stir in the parsley and serve.

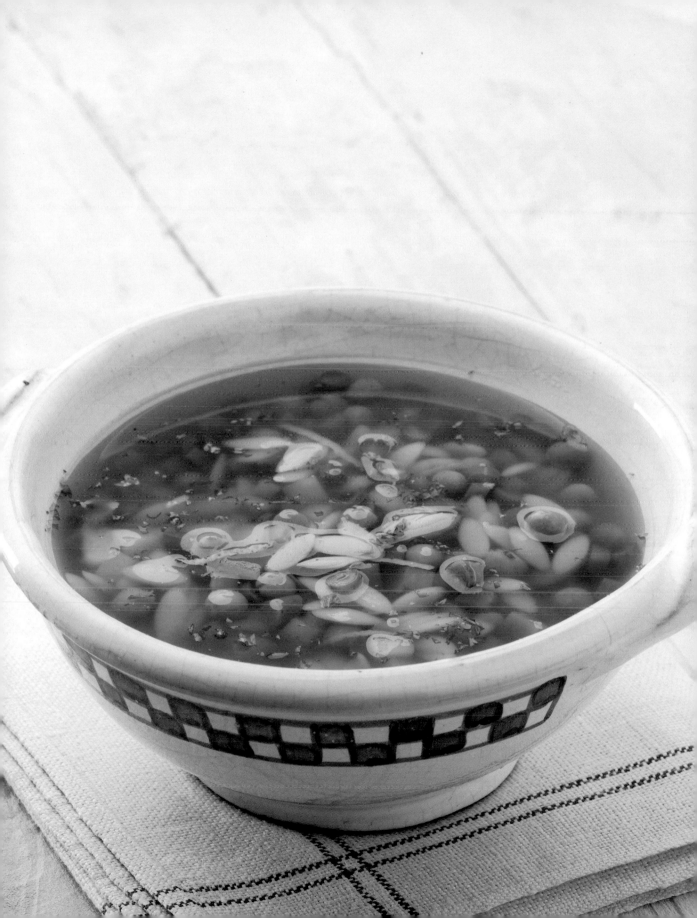

SPRING FARMERS' MARKET SOUP

🗙 🌾 Ⓥ

PREPARATION TIME 15 minutes, plus making the stock

COOKING TIME 35 minutes

1.4l/48fl oz/6 cups Vegetable Stock (see page 12) or ready-made stock

4 large tomatoes, chopped

1 large shallot, sliced

2 large garlic cloves, chopped

1 bouquet garni made with 1 piece of celery stalk with leaves, 1 bay leaf and several basil sprigs tied together

1 tsp sugar

1 tsp dried mint

4 new potatoes, halved or quartered

6 baby carrots, halved lengthways

200g/7oz/1⅓ cups fresh or frozen shelled peas

12 asparagus tips

salt and freshly ground black pepper

freshly grated Parmesan cheese, to serve (optional)

Put the stock, tomatoes, shallot, garlic, bouquet garni and sugar in a saucepan over a high heat. Cover and bring to the boil, then uncover and boil gently for 10 minutes to reduce slightly. Strain the stock into a bowl, pressing down to extract as much flavour as possible.

Return the stock to the pan, add the mint and return to the boil. Add the potatoes and carrots and season with salt and pepper. Reduce the heat and simmer, covered, for 8 minutes. Add the peas and simmer for another 3–5 minutes, if frozen, or for 5–8 minutes, if fresh. Add the asparagus for the final 3 minutes and simmer until all the vegetables are tender but still retain a little crispness. Adjust the salt and pepper, if necessary, and serve with Parmesan cheese on the side, if liked.

SUMMER FARMERS' MARKET SOUP

PREPARATION TIME 15 minutes, plus making the stock and preparing the tomatoes

COOKING TIME 30 minutes

1.4l/48fl oz/6 cups Vegetable Stock (see page 12) or ready-made stock

freshly cut kernels from 2 sweetcorn/corn cobs, with the cobs reserved and halved

1½ tbsp sunflower, olive or hemp oil

1 onion, finely chopped

1 large garlic clove, finely chopped

3 large tomatoes, peeled (see page 10), deseeded and chopped

2 courgettes/zucchini, diced

1½ tsp chopped marjoram leaves

salt and freshly ground black pepper

basil leaves, torn, to serve

Put the stock and corn cobs in a saucepan, season with salt, cover and bring to the boil. Reduce the heat and simmer for 10 minutes, then discard the corn cobs.

Meanwhile, heat the oil in another saucepan over a medium heat. Add the onion and garlic and fry, stirring occasionally, for 3–5 minutes until softened but not coloured. Add the tomatoes and courgettes/zucchini and stir for 2 minutes.

Add the stock and marjoram to the vegetables, cover and bring to the boil. Reduce the heat and simmer for 3 minutes, then add the corn kernels and simmer for another 3–5 minutes until the kernels are tender. Adjust the salt and pepper, if necessary, and serve sprinkled with basil.

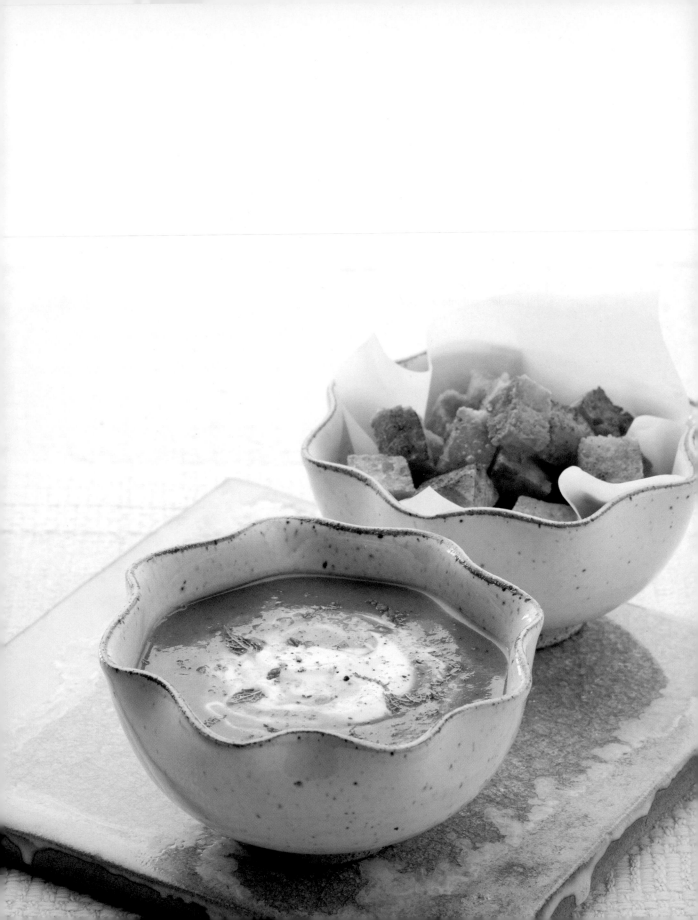

EGYPTIAN AUBERGINE & TOMATO SOUP

(🦐) (V)

PREPARATION TIME 20 minutes, plus making the stock and croûtons (optional)
COOKING TIME 35 minutes

125ml/4fl oz/½ cup olive oil, plus extra as needed

2 aubergines/eggplants (about 700g/1½lb total weight), peeled, cut into 2.5cm/1in slices and patted dry

1 large onion, very finely chopped

2 garlic cloves, very finely chopped

½ tsp ground coriander

½ tsp ground cumin

600ml/20fl oz/2½ cups tomato and vegetable juice

450ml/16fl oz/2 cups Vegetable Stock (see page 12)

6 tbsp Greek-style yogurt

salt and freshly ground black pepper

chopped mint leaves, to serve

1 recipe quantity Garlic Croûtons (see page 18), to serve

Heat two large frying pans over a high heat until a splash of water 'dances' on the surface. Reduce the heat to medium and add a thin layer of oil to each. Add as many aubergine/eggplant slices as will fit in a single layer and fry for 3–3½ minutes on each side until just beginning to brown. Do not overbrown or the soup will taste bitter. Transfer the slices to a large bowl or blender. Add extra oil to the pans between batches, if necessary.

Blend the aubergines/eggplants until smooth, then set aside.

Heat 2 tablespoons of the oil in a saucepan over a medium heat. Add the onion and fry, stirring occasionally, for 10–12 minutes until golden brown. Stir in the garlic, coriander and cumin and fry, stirring continuously, for 30 seconds until aromatic. Add the tomato and vegetable juice and stock, stir in the aubergine/eggplant purée and season with salt and pepper. Cover and bring to the boil, then reduce the heat and simmer, uncovered, for 5 minutes, stirring occasionally.

Stir in the yogurt and adjust the salt and pepper, if necessary. Serve sprinkled with mint and with the croûtons for adding at the table.

TOMATO & THYME SOUP
WITH POLENTA DUMPLINGS

PREPARATION TIME 15 minutes, plus making the stock and dumplings

COOKING TIME 45 minutes

2 tbsp butter

1 tbsp sunflower oil

1 large onion, thinly sliced

1 garlic clove, crushed

175ml/6fl oz/¾ cup dry white wine

3 tbsp plain white/all-purpose or wholemeal/ wholewheat flour

a pinch of mustard powder

600ml/20fl oz/2½ cups Vegetable Stock (see page 12) or ready-made stock

2 cans (800g/1¾lb) chopped tomatoes

½ bunch of lemon thyme, about 15g/½oz, tied together, plus extra leaves to serve

4 tbsp tomato purée/paste

2 tsp caster sugar

240ml/8fl oz/1 cup single/light cream

1 recipe quantity Polenta Dumplings (see page 17)

salt and freshly ground black pepper

Melt the butter with the oil in a saucepan over a medium heat. Add the onion and fry, stirring occasionally, for 2 minutes. Add the garlic and fry for 1–3 minutes until the onion is softened. Stir in the wine, increase the heat to high and cook for 6–8 minutes until almost evaporated, then reduce the heat to low.

Sprinkle in the flour and mustard powder and stir for 2 minutes. Slowly add the stock, stirring to prevent lumps from forming, then stir in the tomatoes, thyme, tomato purée/paste and sugar and season with salt and pepper. Cover and bring to the boil, then reduce the heat and simmer for 15 minutes.

Discard the thyme sprigs and blend the soup. Strain the soup into a large bowl and work it through the sieve, rubbing back and forth with a spoon and scraping the bottom of the sieve. Return the soup to the pan, stir in the cream and reheat without boiling. Add the dumplings and simmer to reheat. Adjust the salt and pepper, if necessary, then serve sprinkled with extra thyme leaves. If you reheat the soup, do not boil it.

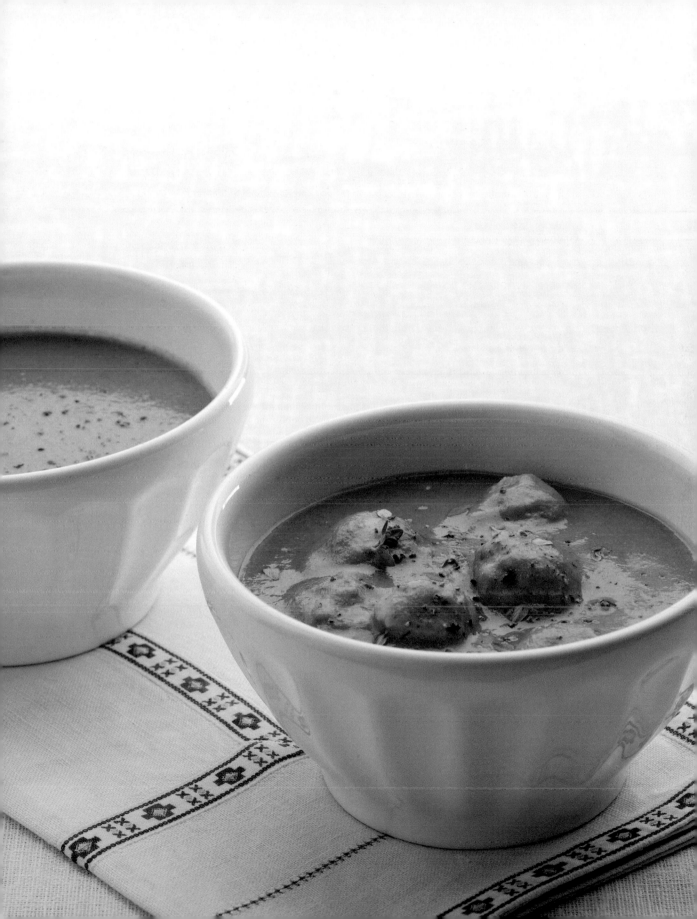

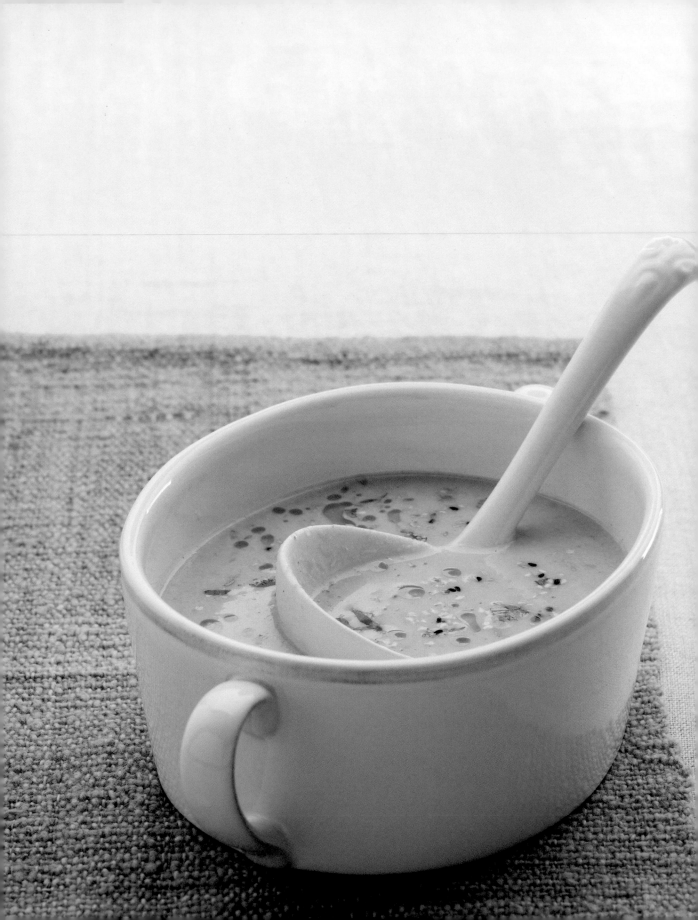

GOLDEN CARROT & SESAME SOUP

PREPARATION TIME 15 minutes, plus making the stock and toasted seeds

COOKING TIME 30 minutes

1½ tbsp olive or hemp oil, plus extra to serve

1 onion, chopped

2 large garlic cloves, chopped

½ tsp ground coriander

¼ tsp turmeric

a pinch of cayenne pepper, or to taste

950ml/32fl oz/4 cups Vegetable Stock (see page 12) or ready-made stock

350g/12oz/2½ cups peeled and thinly sliced carrots

2 tbsp tahini

lemon juice, to taste

salt and freshly ground black pepper

TO SERVE

white sesame seeds, toasted (see page 10)

black sesame seeds

chopped coriander/cilantro leave

Heat the oil in a saucepan over a medium heat. Add the onion and fry, stirring occasionally, for 2 minutes. Add the garlic and fry for 1–3 minutes until the onion is softened but not coloured. Add the ground coriander, turmeric and cayenne pepper and stir for 30 seconds. Watch closely so the spices do not burn.

Add the stock and carrots and season with salt and pepper. Cover and bring to the boil, then reduce the heat and simmer for 12–15 minutes until the carrots are very tender. Add the tahini and stir until it dissolves.

Blend the soup to the preferred consistency, then add the lemon juice and adjust the salt and pepper, if necessary. Serve sprinkled with sesame seeds and coriander/cilantro leaves and drizzled with oil

RED RICE & WILD ROCKET SOUP

PREPARATION TIME 10 minutes, plus making the stock

COOKING TIME 55 minutes

1.5l/52fl oz/6½ cups Vegetable Stock (see page 12) or ready-made stock

4 large garlic cloves, crushed

1 tsp fennel seeds

1½ tbsp olive or hemp oil, plus extra to serve (optional)

2 shallots, halved lengthways and thinly sliced

100g/3½oz/½ cup red rice

1 tsp dried thyme leaves

2 large handfuls of wild rocket/arugula leaves, rinsed and torn

salt and freshly ground black pepper

French bread, to serve

Put the stock, garlic and fennel seeds in a saucepan. Cover and bring to the boil, then boil slowly for 10 minutes to blend the flavours. Strain the stock, discarding the garlic and seeds, and set aside.

Heat the oil in a saucepan over a medium heat. Add the shallots and fry, stirring occasionally, for 3–5 minutes until softened but not coloured. Stir in the rice, then add the stock and thyme and season with salt and pepper. Cover and bring to the boil. Reduce the heat and simmer for 20–25 minutes, or according to the package instructions, until the rice is tender but chewy.

Add the rocket/arugula and simmer, uncovered, for 2–3 minutes until wilted. Adjust the salt and pepper, if necessary, and serve with slices of French bread.

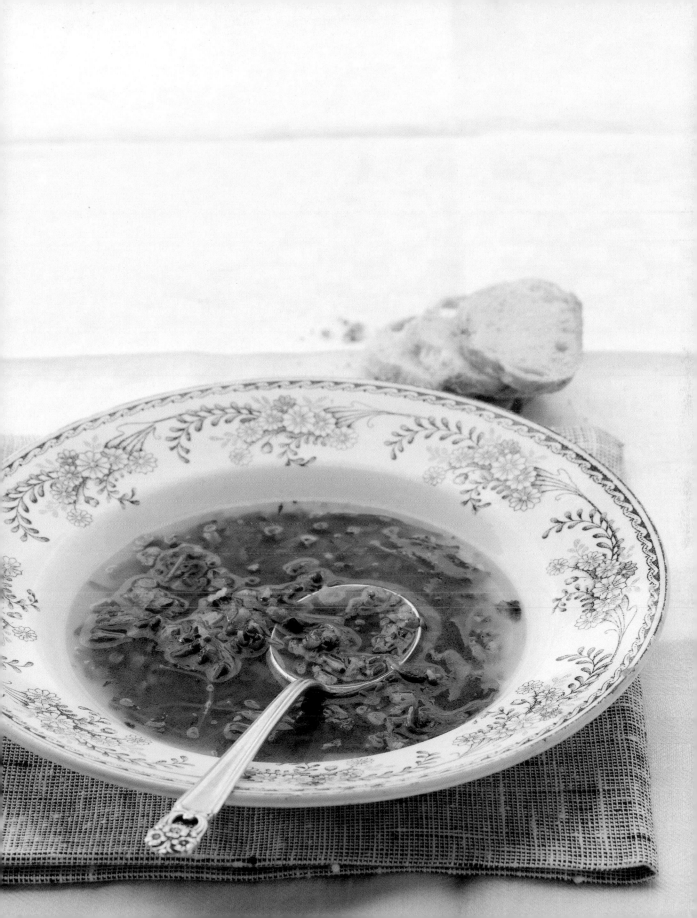

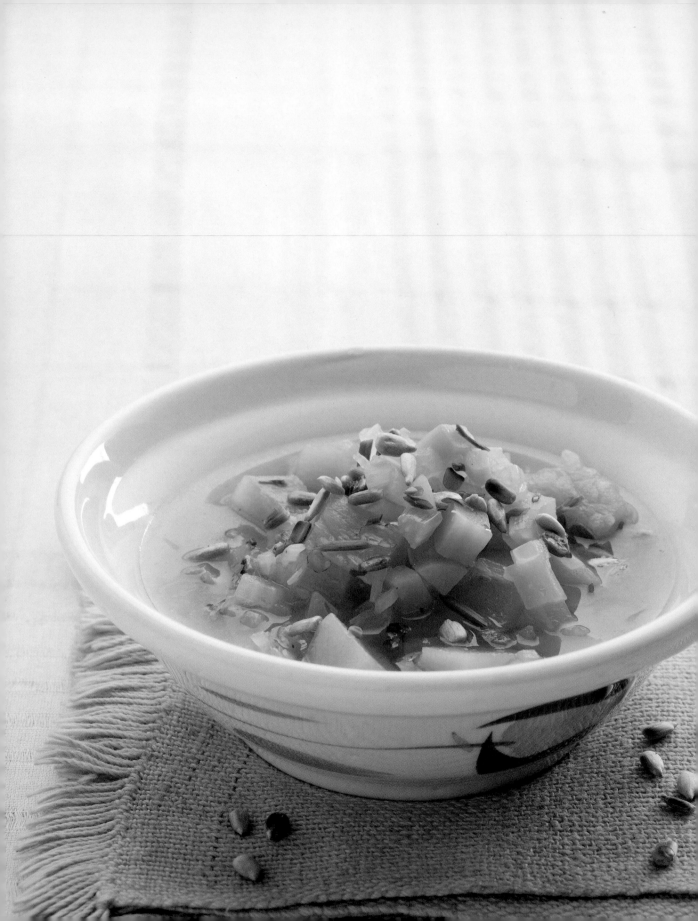

SUNSHINE WINTER SOUP

PREPARATION TIME 15 minutes, plus making the stock and seeds

COOKING TIME 30 minutes

1½ tbsp olive or hemp oil

3 celery stalks, finely chopped, with the leaves reserved

2 large carrots, peeled and diced

2 shallots, finely chopped

1 tsp fennel seeds

a large pinch of saffron threads

1.4l/48fl oz/6 cups Vegetable Stock (see page 12) or ready-made stock

400g/14oz/4 cups peeled, deseeded and diced pumpkin

1 bouquet garni made with the reserved celery leaves, 2 parsley sprigs, 1 bay leaf and 1 thyme sprig tied together

salt and freshly ground black pepper

sunflower seeds, toasted (see page 10), to serve

chopped chives, to serve

Heat the oil in a saucepan over a medium heat. Add the celery, carrots and shallots and stir for 3–5 minutes until the shallots are softened but not coloured. Add the fennel seeds and saffron and stir for 30 seconds until aromatic. Watch closely so they do not burn.

Add the stock, pumpkin and bouquet garni and season with salt and pepper. Cover and bring to the boil, then reduce the heat and simmer, partially covered, for 12–15 minutes until the vegetables are tender. Discard the bouquet garni and adjust the salt and pepper, if necessary. Serve sprinkled with the seeds and chives.

FRENCH ONION SOUP

PREPARATION TIME 10 minutes, plus making the stock and croûtes

COOKING TIME 40 minutes

2 tbsp butter

2 tbsp olive oil

4 large onions, thinly sliced

4 garlic cloves, crushed

1 tsp sugar

1.25l/44fl oz/5½ cups Beef Stock (see page 11) or ready-made stock

6 tbsp brandy

1 bouquet garni made with 1 piece of celery stalk, 1 bay leaf, 4 parsley sprigs and 4 thyme sprigs tied together

salt and freshly ground black pepper

1 Croûte (see page 17) for each bowl, to serve

250g/9oz/2½ cups grated Gruyère cheese, to serve

Melt the butter with the oil in a saucepan over a medium heat. Add the onions and fry, stirring, for 3–5 minutes until softened. Reduce the heat to very low (use a heat diffuser if you have one), stir in the garlic and sugar and fry, stirring frequently, for another 5–8 minutes until the onions are golden brown and caramelized. Add the stock, brandy and bouquet garni and season with salt and pepper. Cover and bring to the boil, then reduce the heat and simmer for 15 minutes.

Meanwhile, preheat the grill/broiler to high. Arrange four or six flameproof soup bowls on a baking sheet and put 1 croûte in each.

Discard the bouquet garni. Ladle the soup into the bowls and divide the cheese over the tops. Grill/broil for 2–3 minutes until the cheese has melted and is bubbling. Serve immediately.

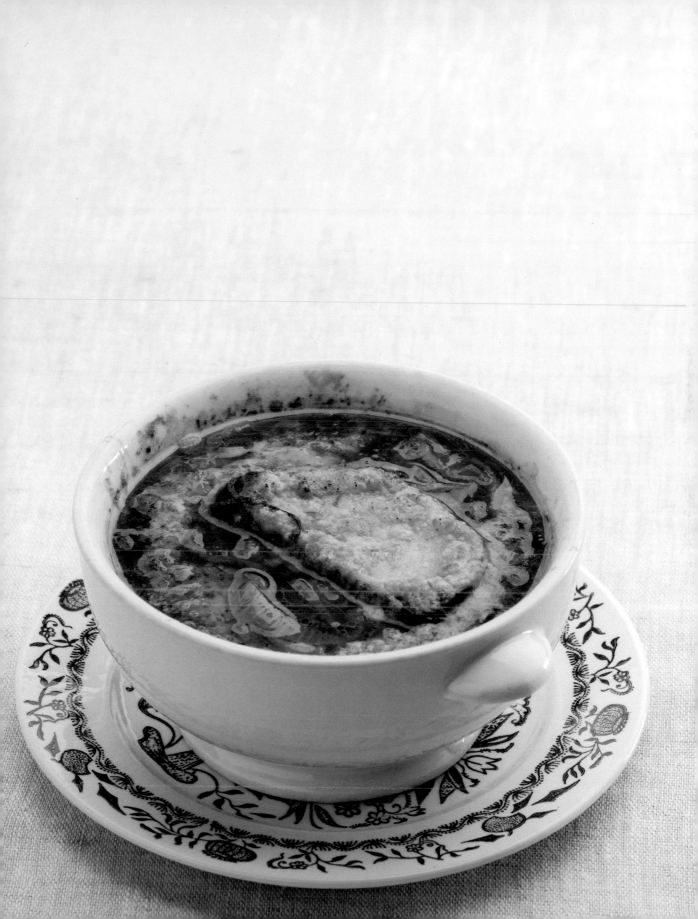

ROASTED SQUASH & TOMATO SOUP

PREPARATION TIME 20 minutes, plus making the stock

COOKING TIME 25 minutes

3 large tomatoes, halved

1 butternut squash (about 600g/1lb 5oz), unpeeled, cut in half, seeds removed and reserved

6 large whole garlic cloves, peeled

1 red onion, quartered

1cm/½in piece of fresh ginger, peeled and thinly sliced

2½ tbsp olive or hemp oil, plus extra for frying the seeds

½ tsp ground coriander

½ tsp ground cumin

½ tsp hot paprika, or to taste

750ml/26fl oz/3¼ cups Vegetable Stock (see page 12) or ready-made stock

salt and freshly ground black pepper

chopped parsley leaves, to serve

Preheat the oven to 220°C/425°F/Gas 7. Put the tomatoes, cut-sides down, in a baking tray. Coarsely chop the squash into 5cm/2in pieces and add it to the baking tray, along with the garlic, onion and ginger. Add the oil, coriander, cumin and paprika and season with salt and pepper. Toss well to coat, then roast for 20 minutes, stirring once or twice, until the squash and onion are tender and the tomato skins have burst.

Meanwhile, put several layers of paper towels on a plate and set aside. Rinse the squash seeds well and use your fingers to remove the fibres, then pat dry with paper towels. Heat a thin layer of the oil in a frying pan over a high heat. Add the seeds and stir for 30 seconds–1 minute until they start to pop and turn golden brown. Watch closely so they do not burn. Immediately turn them out of the pan onto the prepared plate and set aside.

Transfer the vegetables from the baking tray to a large heatproof bowl or blender and add half the stock. Blend until smooth. Working in batches, strain the soup into a saucepan and work it through the sieve, rubbing back and forth with a spoon and scraping the bottom of the sieve. Stir in enough of the remaining stock to achieve the preferred consistency and reheat. (Any leftover stock can be used in other recipes or frozen for up to 6 months.) Adjust the salt and pepper, if necessary, then serve, sprinkled with the seeds and parsley.

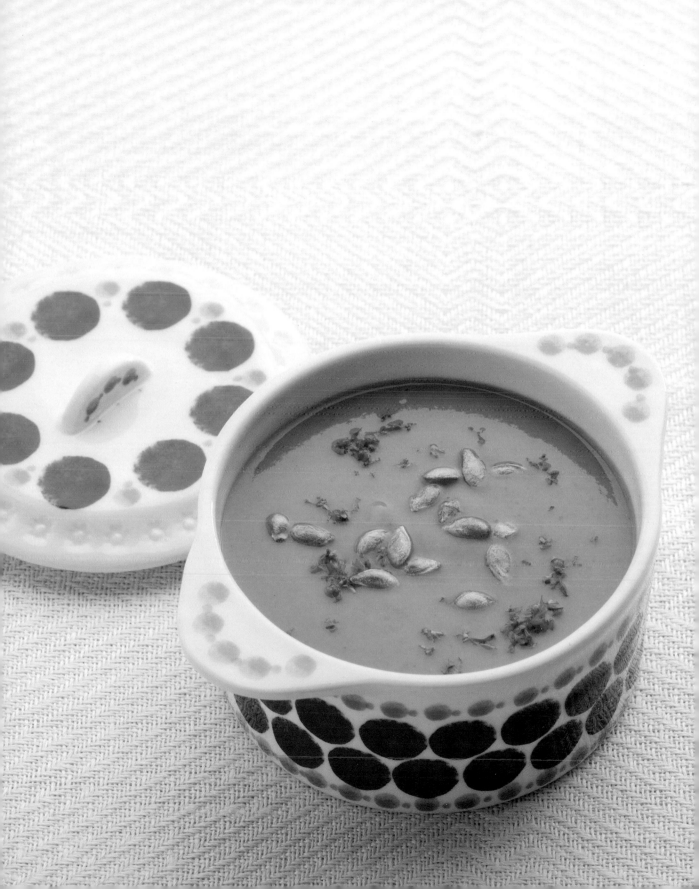

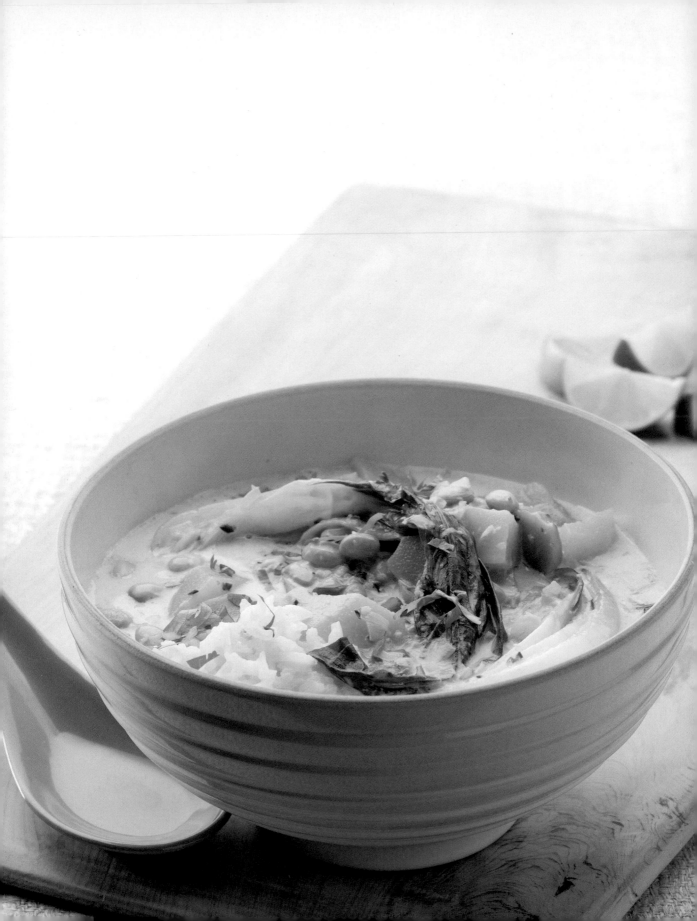

EDAMAME & PUMPKIN SOUP WITH JASMINE RICE

PREPARATION TIME 25 minutes, plus cooking the rice

COOKING TIME 30 minutes

2 tbsp hemp or sunflower oil

1 onion, chopped

2 carrots, peeled and sliced

450g/1lb/3½ cups peeled, deseeded and chopped pumpkin

800ml/28fl oz/3½ cups coconut milk

125g/4½oz/1 cup frozen shelled edamame beans (green soybeans)

4 pak choi/bok choy, quartered lengthways

salt and freshly ground black pepper

280g/10oz/2 cups cooked Thai Jasmine Rice, hot, to serve

chopped coriander/cilantro leaves, to serve

lime wedges, to serve

RED CHILLI PASTE

5 garlic cloves, chopped

2.5cm/1in piece of fresh ginger, peeled and chopped

2 red chillies, deseeded (optional) and chopped

2 lemongrass sticks, chopped, with outer leaves removed

Put all the ingredients for the chilli paste and 2 tablespoons water in a mini food processor and process for 20–30 seconds until a thin, coarse paste forms.

Heat the oil in a heavy stockpot over a high heat. Add the onion and fry, stirring occasionally, for 3–5 minutes until softened but not coloured. Add the chilli paste and stir for 2–3 minutes until the fat separates around the edge. Add the carrots, pumpkin and 1l/35fl oz/4½ cups water and season with salt and pepper. Cover and bring to the boil, then reduce the heat and simmer for 10 minutes.

Add the coconut milk, edamame and pak choi/bok choy and simmer, uncovered, for 3–5 minutes until the edamame are tender. Adjust the salt and pepper, if necessary.

Divide the rice into bowls and ladle the soup over it. Serve sprinkled with chopped coriander/cilantro and with lime wedges for squeezing over.

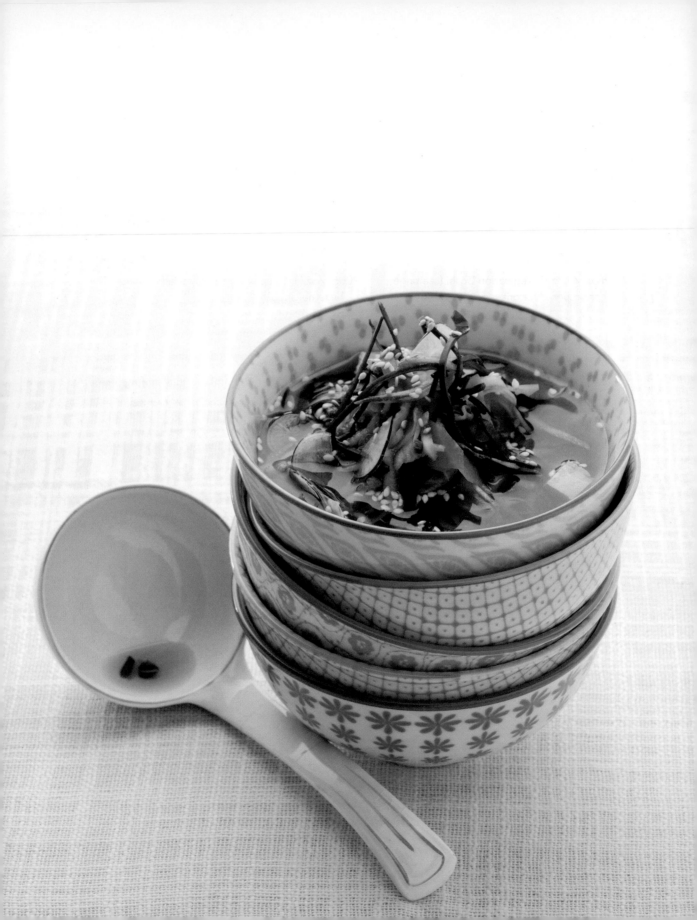

ARAME & TOFU SOUP

PREPARATION TIME 25 minutes, plus making the dashi and seeds

COOKING TIME 15 minutes

20g/¾oz dried arame

1l/35fl oz/4½ cups Vegetarian Dashi (see page 13) or prepared instant vegetarian dashi

2 radishes, very thinly sliced

1 carrot, peeled and coarsely grated

1 red chilli, deseeded and thinly chopped

1 courgette/zucchini, coarsely grated

1 tbsp light soy sauce or tamari soy sauce

1 tbsp rice wine

400g/14oz fried tofu, cut into 1cm/½in cubes

sesame seeds, toasted (see page 10), to serve

Put the arame in a bowl, cover with cold water and leave to soak for 15 minutes until doubled in volume, then drain.

Put the dashi in a saucepan over a high heat, cover and bring to the boil. Add the arame and boil, covered, for 3–5 minutes until tender. Add the radishes, carrot, chilli and courgette/zucchini and boil, uncovered, for 30 seconds–1½ minutes until the vegetables are tender. Stir in the soy sauce and rice wine. Divide the tofu into bowls and ladle the arame and soup over it. Serve sprinkled with sesame seeds.

AUTUMN FARMERS' MARKET SOUP

PREPARATION TIME 15 minutes, plus making the stock and croûtes

COOKING TIME 40 minutes

1½ tbsp olive or hemp oil

200g/7oz/1½ cups deseeded, peeled and diced butternut squash

1 carrot, peeled and diced

2 garlic cloves, finely chopped

1 leek, halved lengthways, thinly sliced and rinsed

300ml/10fl oz/1¼ cups sweet or dry/hard cider

950ml/32fl oz/4 cups Vegetable Stock (see page 12) or ready-made stock

2 sage sprigs

2 tbsp crème fraîche or sour cream (optional)

salt and freshly ground black pepper

chopped parsley leaves, to serve

1 recipe quantity Cheddar Croûtes (see page 17), to serve (optional)

Heat the oil in a saucepan over a medium heat. Stir in the squash, carrot, garlic and leek, cover and reduce the heat to low. Cook for 10–12 minutes, stirring occasionally, until the vegetables begin to soften. Stir in the cider, stock and sage and season, then cover again and bring to the boil.

Reduce the heat and simmer for 15–20 minutes until the vegetables are tender. Discard the sage sprigs, then stir in the crème fraîche, if using. Adjust the salt and pepper, if necessary, and serve sprinkled with parsley and with croûtes on the side, if wished.

HALLOWEEN BEAN SOUP

PREPARATION TIME 15 minutes, plus overnight soaking and cooking the beans (optional), making the stock and toasting the seeds

COOKING TIME 30 minutes

100g/3½oz/½ cup dried black beans or 200g/7oz canned black beans, drained and rinsed

1 tbsp hemp or olive oil

1 large red onion, quartered and thinly sliced

2 large garlic cloves, chopped

1.25l/44fl oz/5½ cups Vegetable Stock (see page 12) or ready-made stock

2 bay leaves

a pinch of dried chilli/hot pepper flakes, or to taste

1 Parmesan or Cheddar cheese rind, about 7.5 x 5cm/3 x 2in (see page 9; optional)

400g/14oz/4 cups peeled, deseeded and chopped pumpkin

2 handfuls of baby spinach leaves

salt and freshly ground black pepper

white sesame seeds, toasted (see page 10), to serve

black sesame seeds, to serve

chopped parsley leaves, to serve

If using dried beans, put them in a bowl, cover with water and leave to soak overnight, then drain and rinse. Transfer to a saucepan, add 1.5l/52fl oz/6½ cups water, cover and bring to the boil. Reduce the heat and simmer, covered, for 50 minutes–1 hour, then drain.

Heat the oil in a saucepan over a medium heat. Add the onion and fry, stirring, for 2 minutes. Add the garlic and stir for 1–3 minutes until the onion is softened. Add the stock, bay leaves, chilli/hot pepper flakes and cheese rind, if using, and season with salt and pepper. Cover and bring to the boil. Add the pumpkin, reduce the heat to medium and simmer for 5–8 minutes until tender.

Add the beans and heat through for 3 minutes. Stir in the spinach and simmer for 1–2 minutes until it wilts. Discard the cheese rind, if used. Adjust the salt and pepper, if necessary, and serve sprinkled with sesame seeds and parsley.

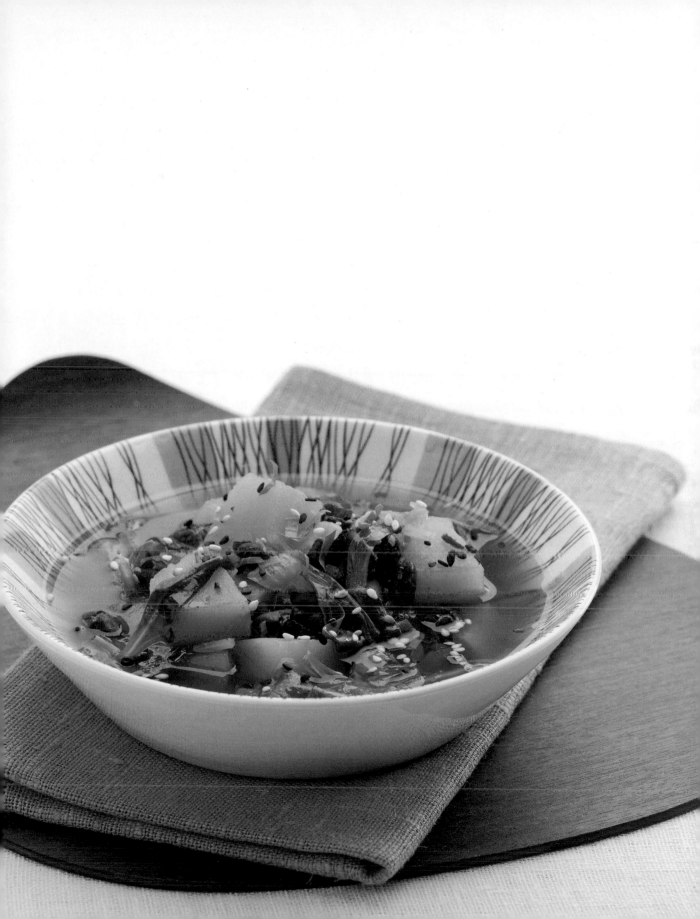

MIXED GRAIN & RED LENTIL SOUP

PREPARATION TIME 10 minutes, plus making the stock and preparing the tomatoes
COOKING TIME 50 minutes

1 tbsp olive or hemp oil

1 large onion, finely chopped

2 large garlic cloves, chopped

1.4l/48fl oz/6 cups Vegetable Stock (see page 12) or ready-made stock

4 tbsp split red lentils, rinsed

2 tbsp bulgar wheat

2 tbsp long-grain white rice

3 tomatoes, grated (see page 10)

1 tbsp dried mint, plus extra to serve

2 tbsp tomato purée/paste

½ tbsp hot or sweet paprika, or to taste

½ tsp cayenne pepper, or to taste

salt and freshly ground black pepper

extra-virgin olive oil, to serve

Heat the oil in a saucepan over a medium heat. Add the onion and fry, stirring, for 2 minutes. Add the garlic and fry for 1–3 minutes until the onion is softened but not coloured. Add the stock, lentils, bulgar wheat, rice, tomatoes, mint, tomato purée/paste, paprika and cayenne. Cover and bring to the boil, then reduce the heat and simmer for 30–40 minutes until the lentils, wheat and rice are all tender. Stir occasionally to prevent the grains from sticking to the base of the pan.

Blend half of the soup until smooth. Return the mixture to the pan, stir well and season with salt and pepper. Serve sprinkled with mint and drizzled with olive oil.

Pictured on page 112

GUJARATI YOGURT SOUP

PREPARATION TIME 15 minutes

COOKING TIME 10 minutes

8 fresh curry leaves

1 green chilli, deseeded (optional) and chopped, or to taste

1cm/½in piece of fresh ginger, peeled and grated, or to taste

5mm/¼in piece of white turmeric (optional)

2.5cm/1in piece of cucumber, deseeded and chopped

2 tbsp gram (chickpea/garbanzo bean) flour

½ tsp ground coriander

600g/1lb 5oz/heaped 2½ cups plain yogurt

2 tbsp ghee or sunflower oil

1 tsp cumin seeds

1 tsp black mustard seeds

½ tsp fenugreek seeds

a pinch of ground asafoetida

salt

2 handfuls of coriander/cilantro leaves, torn

Put half the curry leaves, the chilli, ginger and white turmeric, if using, in a small food processor and blend until very finely chopped (or use a mortar and pestle). Add the cucumber and blend again until the mixture forms a paste.

Put the gram flour and ground coriander in a bowl and season with salt, then add the yogurt and 600ml/20fl oz/2½ cups water and stir until smooth. Adjust the salt, if necessary, adding more chilli and ginger, if you like.

Melt the ghee in a saucepan over a medium heat. Add the cumin, mustard and fenugreek seeds and stir for 30 seconds until they crackle and pop. Watch closely so they do not burn. Stir in the asafoetida and remaining curry leaves and stir just until the leaves sizzle.

Reduce the heat to very low (use a heat diffuser if you have one) and add the yogurt mixture, stirring continuously to prevent it from separating. Watch closely because the mixture will splutter. Stir for 8–10 minutes until the soup thickens. Serve sprinkled with the coriander/cilantro leaves.

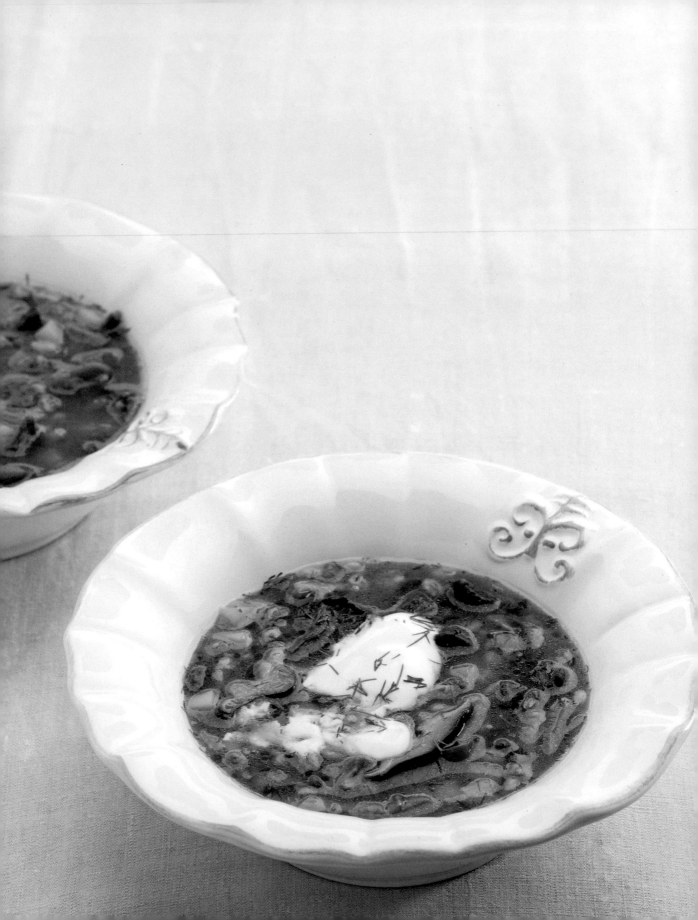

WILD MUSHROOM &
TOASTED SPELT SOUP

PREPARATION TIME 15 minutes, plus 30 minutes soaking the mushrooms and making the stock

COOKING TIME 1 hour

30g/1oz dried porcini mushrooms

2 tbsp olive or hemp oil

85g/3oz/½ cup spelt

1 tbsp butter

1 celery stalk, finely chopped,
with the leaves reserved

1 large red onion, finely chopped

400g/14oz/4½ cups trimmed and coarsely
chopped mixed wild mushrooms, such as
chanterelles, horns of plenty and oysters

2 large garlic cloves, chopped

1l/35fl oz/4½ cups Beef Stock (see page 11)
or ready-made stock

1 bouquet garni made with the celery leaves,
1 bay leaf and several parsley and thyme sprigs
tied together

1 large waxy potato, diced

1 small handful of dill, finely chopped

salt and freshly ground black pepper

sour cream or smetana, to serve

Put the porcini mushrooms and at least 200ml/
7fl oz/scant 1 cup boiling water in a heatproof
bowl and leave to soak for 30 minutes until
tender. Strain through a muslin-lined/cheesecloth-
lined sieve and set the liquid aside. Squeeze the
mushrooms and trim the stalks, if necessary, then
thinly slice the caps and stalks and set aside.

Heat 1 tablespoon of the oil in a saucepan over
a high heat. Add the spelt and stir for 2–3 minutes
until it gives off a toasted aroma. Immediately
transfer to a bowl and set aside.

Melt the butter with the remaining oil in the pan
over a medium heat. Add the celery and onion
and fry, stirring, for 2 minutes. Stir in the wild
mushrooms and garlic, season with salt and fry
for 5–8 minutes, stirring occasionally, until the
mushrooms soften and give off their liquid.

Stir in the spelt and fry for 2 minutes, then add
the stock, bouquet garni, porcini mushrooms and
reserved soaking liquid and season with salt and
pepper. Cover and bring to the boil. Reduce the
heat and simmer for 20 minutes, then stir in the
potato and simmer for 15–20 minutes until the
spelt and potato are tender. Stir in the dill and
adjust the salt and pepper, if necessary. Serve
with sour cream.

BEETROOT & APPLE SOUP

PREPARATION TIME 15 minutes, plus making the stock

COOKING TIME 55 minutes

1 large cooking apple, peeled and chopped

1 tbsp lemon juice

1½ tbsp olive or hemp oil

1 onion, chopped

½ tbsp caraway seeds

800ml/28fl oz/3½ cups Vegetable Stock (see page 12)

450g/1lb/3½ cups peeled and diced beetroots/beets

salt and freshly ground black pepper

HORSERADISH & DILL CREAM

5 tbsp sour cream

1 tbsp grated horseradish

½ tbsp chopped dill, plus extra to serve

a pinch of salt

Toss the apple and lemon juice together in a bowl and set aside. Heat the oil in a saucepan over a medium heat. Add the onion and fry, stirring, for 3–5 minutes until softened. Add the caraway seeds and stir for 30 seconds until aromatic. Watch closely so they do not burn. Add the stock and beetroot/beets, cover and bring to the boil. Reduce the heat and simmer for 30 minutes.

Meanwhile, make the horseradish and dill cream. Put all the ingredients in a bowl and stir, then cover and chill.

Add the apple and any remaining lemon juice to the pan and simmer for another 10 minutes until the beetroots/beets are tender. Blend the soup until smooth, then season with salt and pepper. Serve topped with the horseradish cream and an extra sprinkling of dill.

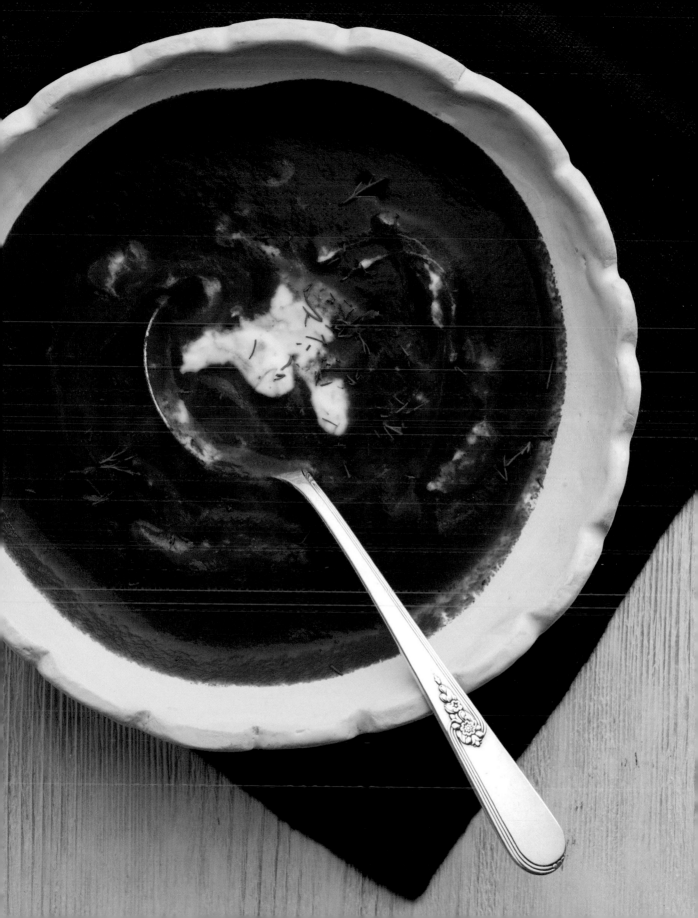

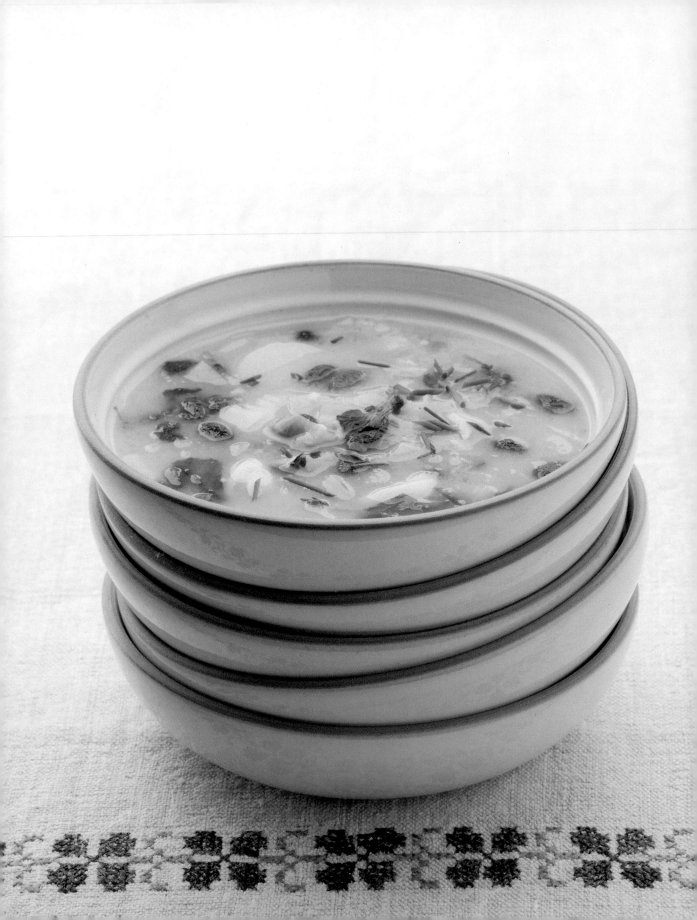

GOJI BERRY & GARLIC SOUP

PREPARATION TIME 15 minutes, plus making the stock

COOKING TIME 35 minutes

1.5l/52fl oz/6½ cups Rich Chicken Stock
(see page 11), Chicken Stock (see page 12)
or Vegetable Stock (see page 12)

1 large garlic bulb, separated into cloves

2 leeks, halved lengthways, sliced and rinsed

1cm/½in piece of fresh ginger, peeled and grated

a pinch of dried chilli/hot pepper flakes,
or to taste

grated zest of 1 lemon

2 tbsp medium rolled oats

1 tbsp honey

2–4 tbsp lemon juice

2 tbsp dried goji berries

1 large handful of watercress leaves, torn

chopped chives, to serve

Put the stock and garlic in a saucepan, cover and bring to the boil. Boil for 15 minutes until the garlic is very tender. Use a fork to mash the garlic against the side of the pan, then stir in the leeks, ginger, chilli/hot pepper flakes, lemon zest and oats. Reduce the heat and simmer, covered, for 8–10 minutes until thickened slightly and the oats are tender.

Stir in the honey and 1 tablespoon of the lemon juice, then add the remaining juice to taste. Stir in the goji berries and watercress and simmer, uncovered, for 1 minute until the berries are softened. Serve sprinkled with chives.

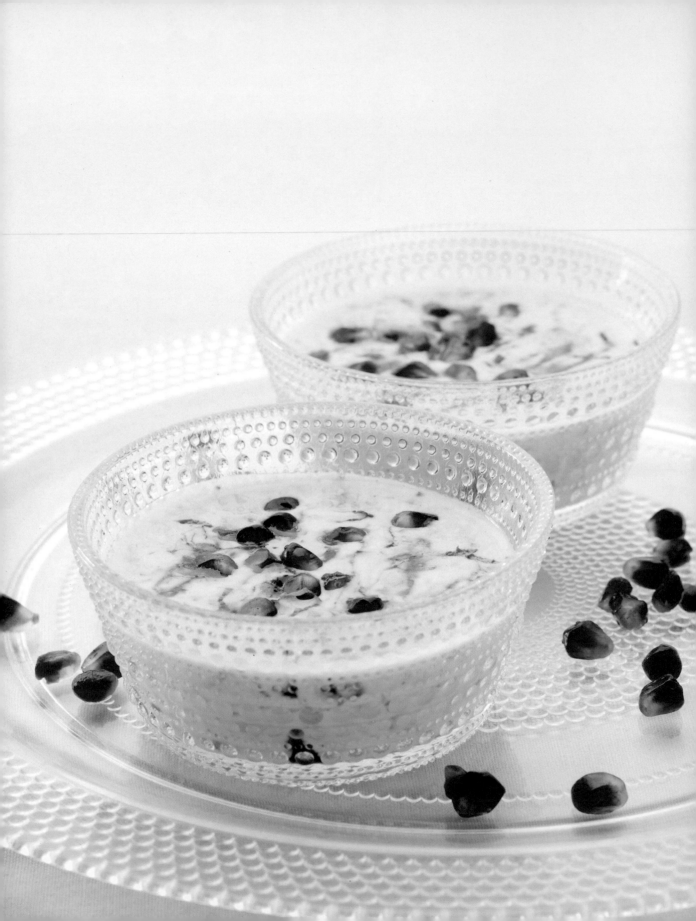

CHILLED SOUPS

The sweet and savoury soups in this chapter are the key to staying cool in the kitchen when temperatures are high. These recipes include meat- and chicken-based soups, as well as vegetarian and vegan options.

From sunny Spain, Gazpacho and White Garlic & Almond Soup are ideal for summer entertaining, as is Bloody Mary Party Soup. And, if rain clouds threaten your catering plans, don't worry: Fennel & Red Pepper Soups, Consommé & Vegetable Soup and Lemon & Saffron Soup can do double duty as hot soups.

The important thing to remember with the recipes in this chapter is to taste and adjust the seasoning with salt and pepper, if necessary, before serving. Chilling soups dulls the flavours, and what previously tasted fresh and exciting might need re-seasoning after several hours in the refrigerator. Most soups also thicken as they chill and will require a little extra liquid stirred in just before serving.

GAZPACHO

PREPARATION TIME 20 minutes, plus preparing the tomatoes,
at least 2 hours chilling and making the croûtons

6 large tomatoes, peeled (see page 10),
deseeded and chopped

2 red peppers, deseeded and chopped

2 large garlic cloves, coarsely chopped

400g/14oz/3 cups peeled, deseeded and
chopped cucumber

4 tbsp extra-virgin olive oil, plus extra to serve

tomato juice (optional)

sherry vinegar, to taste

salt and freshly ground black pepper

TO SERVE

1 recipe quantity Garlic Croûtons (see page 18)

2 spring onions/scallions, thinly sliced

1 large green pepper, deseeded and finely diced

1 large red pepper, deseeded and finely diced

½ cucumber, peeled, deseeded and finely diced

ice cubes (optional)

Blend the tomatoes, peppers, garlic, cucumber and oil to the preferred consistency. Depending on how juicy the tomatoes were, it might be necessary to stir in a little tomato juice to give the soup a more liquid texture. Strain the soup for an even smoother texture, if you like.

Season with salt and pepper, add sherry vinegar and blend again. Cover and chill for at least 2 hours.

When ready to serve, stir well. Adjust the salt and pepper and add more vinegar, if necessary. Serve with an ice cube added to each portion, if you like, and with the croûtons, spring onions/ scallions, peppers and cucumber on the side.

CONSOMMÉ & VEGETABLE SOUP

PREPARATION TIME 15 minutes, plus making the consommé, preparing the tomato, cooling and at least 2 hours chilling

1 carrot, peeled and grated

1 courgette/zucchini, peeled and grated

1 tomato, peeled (see page 10), deseeded and finely diced

2 tbsp finely chopped chives

2 tbsp finely chopped parsley leaves

1 recipe quantity Beef or Chicken Consommé (see pages 13 and 14) or 1.25l/44fl oz/ 5½ cups canned beef or chicken consommé, at room temperature

salt and freshly ground black pepper

dry sherry, to serve

1 pomegranate, to serve (optional)

Put the carrot, courgette/zucchini, tomato, chives, parsley and consommé in a bowl, stir well and season very lightly with salt and pepper. Cover and chill for at least 2 hours. The consommé will lightly gel while chilling.

When ready to serve, put 1 teaspoon dry sherry in each bowl, then ladle in the soup. If you want to garnish with pomegranate seeds, bash the pomegranate with a wooden spoon, then cut it in half. Hold one half over one of the bowls and tap the top with the spoon so the seeds fall over the soup and remove any white pith. Repeat to sprinkle the remaining bowls with pomegranate seeds, then serve.

CREAMY COURGETTE SOUP

PREPARATION TIME 15 minutes, plus making the stock, cooling and at least 2 hours chilling

COOKING TIME 20 minutes

875ml/30fl oz/3¾ cups Vegetable Stock (see page 12) or ready-made stock, plus extra as needed

350g/12oz/2½ cups sliced courgettes/zucchini

1 onion, chopped

175g/6oz/¾ cup soft garlic-and-herb cream cheese

salt and ground white pepper

2 tbsp finely chopped parsley leaves, to serve

Put the stock, courgettes/zucchini and onion in a saucepan. Season with salt and white pepper, cover and bring to the boil. Reduce the heat and simmer for 8–10 minutes until the courgettes/ zucchini are very tender, then blend until smooth.

Put the cheese in a small bowl, add several spoonfuls of the soup and beat until smooth. Add this mixture to the soup, stirring until well blended. Set aside and leave to cool completely, then cover and chill for at least 2 hours.

When ready to serve, add a little extra stock if the soup has thickened. Adjust the salt and pepper, if necessary, and serve sprinkled with parsley.

BLOODY MARY PARTY SOUP

PREPARATION TIME 15 minutes, plus making the stock, cooling and at least 2 hours chilling

COOKING TIME 30 minutes

MAKES 14 x 100ml/3½fl oz/scant ½ cup servings or 4–6 conventional servings

1 tbsp chilli-flavoured olive oil

100g/3½oz/¾ cup peeled and diced carrot

1 celery stalk, finely chopped, plus extra celery stalks with leaves to serve (optional)

1 onion, finely chopped

700ml/24fl oz/3 cups passata (Italian sieved tomatoes), plus extra as needed

750ml/26fl oz/3¼ cups Vegetable Stock (see page 12) or ready-made stock, plus extra as needed

150ml/5fl oz/⅔ cup vodka

a pinch of dried chilli/hot pepper flakes, or to taste

lemon juice, to taste

salt and freshly ground black pepper

sweet sherry, to serve

celery salt, to serve

celery seeds, to serve

Heat the oil in a saucepan over a medium heat. Stir in the carrot, celery and onion, reduce the heat to low and cook, covered, for 8–10 minutes, stirring occasionally, until softened. Stir in the passata, stock, vodka and chilli/hot pepper flakes and season with salt and pepper. Cover and bring to the boil, then reduce the heat and simmer for 10 minutes. Add lemon juice to taste, then blend until smooth.

Strain the soup through a sieve into a large bowl, rubbing back and forth with a spoon and scraping the bottom of the sieve. Set aside to cool completely, then cover and chill for at least 2 hours.

When ready to serve, stir the soup and add a little extra passata or stock if it has thickened. Adjust the salt and pepper, if necessary. Put ½ teaspoon sweet sherry in fourteen small or four to six regular mugs or glasses. Add the soup, sprinkle with celery salt and celery seeds, add celery stalks to act as stirrers, if you like, and serve.

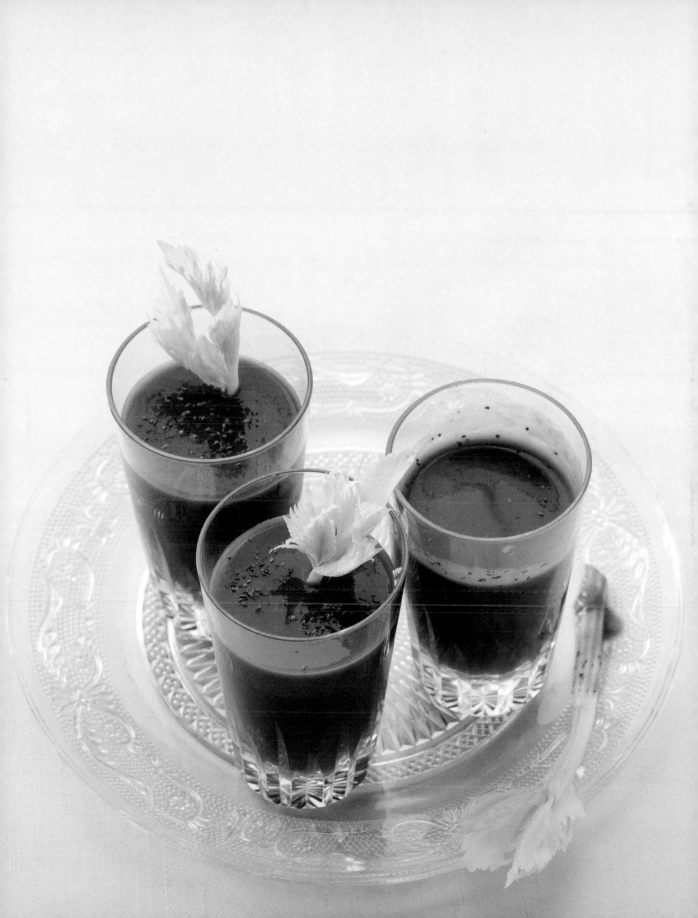

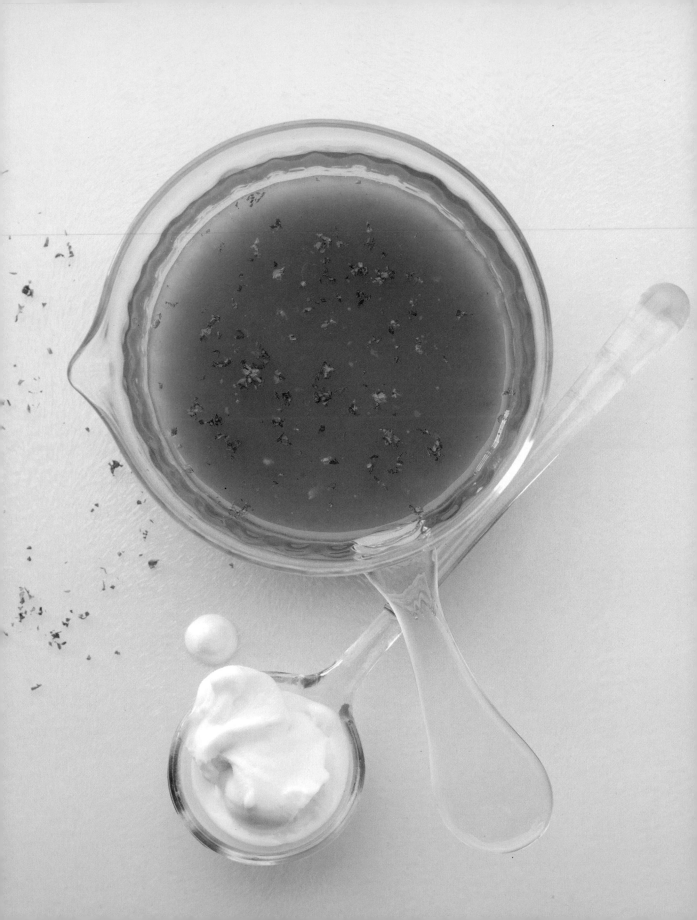

ICED TOMATO & ORANGE SOUP WITH GOATS' MILK-YOGURT SORBET

🐟 🌿 Ⓥ

PREPARATION TIME 5 minutes, plus making, cooling and at least 2 hours chilling the soup and 2 hours freezing the sorbet

COOKING TIME 10 minutes

1 recipe quantity Slow-Cooked Tomato & Orange Soup (see page 118), chilled for at least 2 hours

orange juice (optional)

salt and freshly ground black pepper (optional)

very finely chopped parsley, to serve

GOATS' MILK-YOGURT SORBET

250g/9oz/heaped 1 cup goats' milk yogurt

200g/7oz/1 cup sugar

1 tbsp lemon juice

To make the sorbet, put the yogurt, sugar, lemon juice and 175ml/6fl oz/¾ cup water in a saucepan over a medium heat and stir until the sugar dissolves. Bring to the boil, then boil, without stirring, for 5 minutes. Brush down the side of the pan with a wet pastry brush, if the mixture splashes the side, but do not stir.

Pour the mixture into a shallow heatproof bowl and set aside to cool completely. Churn the sorbet in an ice-cream maker, following the manufacturer's directions, then transfer to a freezerproof bowl and freeze until required. Alternatively, put the mixture in the freezer and freeze for 2 hours. Use an electric mixer or fork to beat the semi-frozen mixture, then return it to the freezer. Repeat two more times, then return the sorbet to the freezer until required.

Remove the sorbet from the freezer 10 minutes before serving. When ready to serve, stir the soup well and add extra orange juice, if you like. Adjust the salt and pepper, if necessary, and serve immediately with 1 scoop of sorbet per portion, sprinkled with parsley. Any leftover sorbet can be kept frozen for up to 3 months.

SPANISH WHITE GARLIC & ALMOND SOUP

V

PREPARATION TIME 15 minutes, plus at least 2 hours freezing the grapes and chilling the water

COOKING TIME 10 minutes

1 small bunch of seedless white grapes, to serve

8 large garlic cloves, peeled but left whole

250g/9oz day-old country-style bread, crusts removed

4–6 tbsp sherry vinegar

250g/9oz/2½ cups ground almonds

125ml/4fl oz/½ cup extra-virgin olive oil, plus extra to serve

salt and ground white pepper

At least 2 hours before serving, put the grapes in the freezer and put a jug with 1.25l/44fl oz/ 5½ cups water in the refrigerator to chill. If your refrigerator is large enough, chill the serving bowls as well.

Put the garlic cloves in a small saucepan and cover with water. Cover and bring to the boil, then strain into a bowl and set the garlic aside. Tear the bread into a large bowl, sprinkle with the garlic-flavoured water and set aside for 10–12 minutes until softened, then use your hands to squeeze any water from the bread.

Blend the bread with the garlic, 4 tablespoons of the vinegar, the ground almonds and the oil to form a thick paste-like mixture. Season with salt and white pepper. Slowly add the chilled water and continue blending to achieve the preferred consistency. Adjust the salt and pepper and add the remaining sherry vinegar, if you like. At this point, the soup can be served as it is, or covered and chilled until required.

When ready to serve, stir well and add extra chilled water if the soup has thickened. Serve with the frozen grapes acting as ice cubes and drizzle with oil.

LEMON & SAFFRON SOUP

V

PREPARATION TIME 10 minutes, plus making the stock, cooling and at least 2 hours chilling

COOKING TIME 45 minutes

1 large lemon, well scrubbed

2 tbsp butter

2 tbsp plain white/all-purpose flour

a large pinch of saffron threads

950ml/32fl oz/4 cups Vegetable Stock (see page 12) or ready-made stock, plus extra as needed

150ml/5fl oz/⅔ cup crème fraîche or sour cream

salt and ground white pepper

finely shredded mint leaves, to serve

goji berries (optional), to serve

Put the lemon in a small saucepan and cover generously with water. Cover and bring to the boil, boil for 5 minutes, then drain. Repeat this process three more times. After the fourth time, cut the lemon in half in a soup bowl to capture all the juices and set aside.

Melt the butter in a large saucepan over a medium heat. Sprinkle in the flour, add the saffron and stir for 2 minutes. Remove the pan from the heat and slowly pour in the stock, stirring continuously to prevent lumps from forming. Stir in the crème fraîche, then return the soup to the heat and bring to the boil, stirring. Boil for 2 minutes, then remove from the heat and set aside.

Use the tip of a knife to remove the seeds from the lemon halves, then chop each half, including the skins. Add the lemon and any accumulated juices to the soup and blend until smooth. Season with salt and white pepper. Set aside to cool completely, then cover and chill for at least 2 hours.

When ready to serve, add a little extra stock if the soup has thickened and stir well. Adjust the salt and pepper, if necessary, and serve sprinkled with mint leaves and goji berries, if you like. This soup is also good served hot, sprinkled with mint leaves and chopped pistachio nuts.

FENNEL & RED PEPPER SOUPS

PREPARATION TIME 25 minutes, plus making the stock, cooling and at least 2 hours chilling
COOKING TIME 40 minutes

4 tbsp olive oil

2 onions, very finely chopped

2 fennel bulbs, finely chopped, with the fronds reserved and chopped

125ml/4fl oz/½ cup Vegetable Stock (see page 12) or ready-made stock

2 tbsp lemon juice

1 tsp aniseed-flavoured spirit, such as Pernod

2 large red peppers, deseeded and diced

a pinch of cayenne pepper

1 tbsp crème fraîche or sour cream

salt and ground white pepper

Heat the oil in a saucepan over a medium heat. Add the onions and fry, stirring occasionally, for 3–5 minutes until softened. Remove half the onions and set aside.

To make the fennel soup, add the fennel to the onion in the pan and cook, stirring, for 5 minutes. Add half the stock, the lemon juice, spirit and enough water to cover. Season with salt and white pepper. Cover and bring to the boil, then reduce the heat and simmer for 12–15 minutes until the fennel is very tender.

Blend until smooth, then work the soup through a sieve into a bowl. Stir in the crème fraîche and set aside to cool completely, then cover and chill for at least 2 hours.

Meanwhile, make the red pepper soup. Put the remaining onion in a saucepan and reheat. Add the peppers and cook, stirring, for 5 minutes. Add the remaining stock, cayenne pepper and enough water to cover, and season with salt. Cover and bring to the boil, then reduce the heat and simmer for 12–15 minutes until the peppers are very tender. Blend until smooth. Work the soup through a sieve into a bowl. Set aside to cool completely, then cover and chill for at least 2 hours.

To serve, stir each soup and adjust the salt and pepper, if necessary. Filling one soup bowl at a time, put the fennel soup in half the bowl, then add the red pepper soup to the other half and use the tip of a knife to swirl decoratively.

Alternatively, put a metal ring in the middle and fill it with the fennel soup. Spoon the red pepper soup around the outside of the ring, then carefully lift the ring. In any case, always pour the fennel soup first because it is thicker and will remain in position. Sprinkle with the fennel fronds and serve.

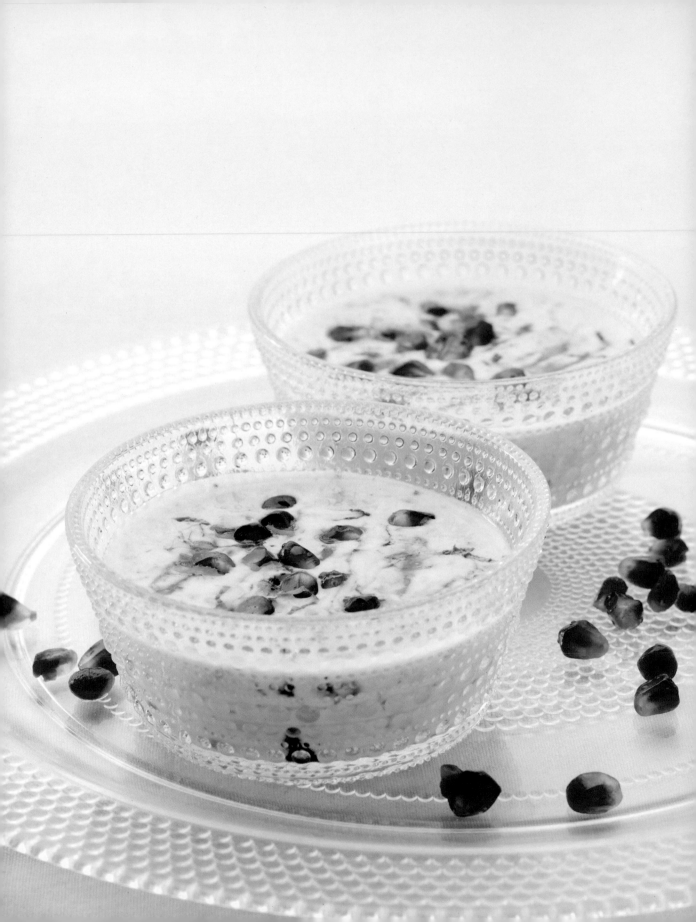

JEWELLED CUCUMBER & WALNUT SOUP

🌾 Ⓥ

PREPARATION TIME 15 minutes, plus making the stock, toasting the walnuts,
30 minutes standing and at least 2 hours chilling

280g/10oz/2 cups grated cucumber

½ tsp salt, plus extra to season

600g/1lb 5oz/2½ cups Greek-style yogurt,
plus extra as needed

600ml/20fl oz/2½ cups Vegetable Stock
(see page 12) or ready-made stock

2 garlic cloves, crushed

85g/3oz/¾ cup walnut halves, very lightly
toasted (see page 10) and finely chopped

2 tbsp finely chopped mint leaves,
plus extra to serve

freshly ground white pepper

pomegranate syrup, to serve

walnut oil, to serve

1 pomegranate, to serve

Put the cucumber in a sieve, sprinkle with the salt and leave to drain for 30 minutes, then rinse under cold running water and pat dry. Transfer the cucumber to a bowl and stir in the yogurt, stock, garlic, walnuts and mint. Season with salt and white pepper, then cover and chill for at least 2 hours.

When ready to serve, stir well and add a little extra yogurt if the soup has thickened. Adjust the salt and pepper, if necessary, and divide into bowls. Sprinkle with mint and drizzle with pomegranate syrup and walnut oil. Bash the pomegranate with a wooden spoon, then cut it in half. Hold one half over one of the bowls and tap the top with the spoon so the seeds fall over the soup. Remove any white pith, if necessary. Repeat to sprinkle the remaining bowls with pomegranate seeds, then serve.

GREEN TEA SOUP WITH COCONUT JELLY

※ Ⓥ

PREPARATION TIME 15 minutes, plus chilling the coconut jelly, cooling the soup and 2 hours chilling
COOKING TIME 15 minutes

2 tbsp matcha (green tea powder)
1.25l/44fl oz/5½ cups whole milk
1 tbsp sugar, or to taste
finely grated lime zest, to serve

COCONUT JELLY
240ml/8fl oz/1 cup coconut milk
1 heaped tbsp agar agar flakes
1 tbsp sugar

To make the coconut jelly, rinse the inside of a shallow, heatproof 8.5 x 12cm/3½ x 4½in dish (or use a small ice cube tray), then pour the water out, but do not dry it, and set aside. Put the coconut milk, agar agar flakes and sugar in a saucepan. Bring to a simmer over a low heat, without stirring. Once it is simmering, stir occasionally for 3–5 minutes until the agar agar flakes dissolve completely – put some of the mixture in a clean spoon and look closely for any specks of agar agar. Pour the mixture into the prepared dish and set aside to cool completely. Cover and chill to set while you make the soup.

Mix the matcha and a little of the milk together in a small bowl to make a thin paste, then stir the mixture into the rinsed-out saucepan, along with the remaining milk and the sugar. Bring to just below the boil and stir until the sugar has dissolved, then remove the pan from the heat and pour the soup into a heatproof bowl. Set aside to cool completely, then cover and chill for at least 2 hours.

When ready to serve, run the tip of a round-bladed knife around the edges of the coconut jelly, then invert it onto a plate, shake well and remove the dish. Cut the jelly into bite size pieces. Stir the soup and add extra sugar, if you like. Serve topped with the coconut jelly and lime zest.

MINTED PEA SOUP

PREPARATION TIME 15 minutes, plus making the stock, cooling and at least 2 hours chilling

COOKING TIME 30 minutes

1½ tbsp olive or hemp oil, plus extra to serve

4 spring onions/scallions, finely chopped, plus extra, thinly sliced on the diagonal, to serve

1 floury/russet potato, peeled and finely chopped

900ml/32fl oz/4 cups Vegetable Stock (see page 12) or ready-made stock, plus extra as needed

600g/1lb 5oz/4 cups frozen peas

30g/1oz mint leaves, plus extra small ones to serve

salt and freshly ground black pepper

Heat the oil in a saucepan over a medium heat. Add the spring onions/scallions and fry, stirring, for 3–5 minutes until softened but not coloured. Stir in the potato, then add the stock and season with salt and pepper, cover and bring to the boil. Reduce the heat and simmer for 10–12 minutes until the potato is tender. Add the peas and mint, return to the boil, uncovered, then reduce the heat and simmer for 3–5 minutes until the peas are tender.

Blend the soup. For a smoother texture, work it through a sieve, if you like, rubbing back and forth with a spoon and scraping the bottom of the sieve to remove the pea skins. Leave to cool completely, then cover and chill for at least 2 hours.

When ready to serve, stir well and add extra stock if the soup has thickened. Adjust the salt and pepper, if necessary. Serve sprinkled with spring onions/scallions and mint leaves and drizzled with a little olive oil.

HUNGARIAN CHERRY SOUP

🌾 Ⓥ

PREPARATION TIME 15 minutes, plus toasting the almonds, cooling and at least 2 hours chilling

COOKING TIME 20 minutes

900g/2lb fresh cherries, pitted

240ml/8fl oz/1 cup rosé or dry red wine

1 tbsp light brown sugar

1 cinnamon stick

pared zest of 1 large lemon, all bitter white pith removed

175g/6oz/¾ cup Greek-style yogurt, smetana or sour cream

1 tsp almond extract

lemon juice, to taste

salt

2 tbsp cherry brandy or kirsch (optional)

flaked/slivered almonds, toasted (see page 10), to serve

Put the cherries, wine, sugar, cinnamon stick, lemon zest and 200ml/7fl oz/scant 1 cup water in a saucepan and stir to dissolve the sugar. Cover and bring to just below the boil, then reduce the heat and simmer for 10–12 minutes until the cherries are very tender.

Discard the cinnamon stick and lemon zest and blend the soup until smooth. Stir in the yogurt, almond extract and lemon juice and season lightly with salt. Transfer to a bowl and set aside to cool completely, then cover and chill for at least 2 hours.

When ready to serve, stir in the brandy, if using. Adjust the salt and add extra lemon juice, if necessary, then serve sprinkled with almonds, either as a dessert soup or, as in Hungary, as a first course.

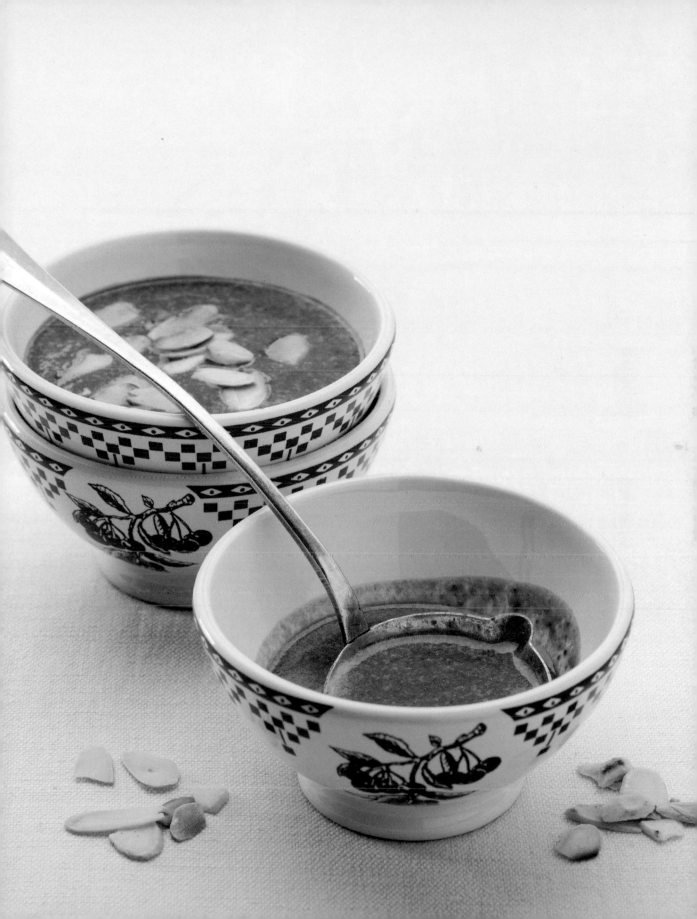

INDEX